THE NLN JEFFRIES SIMULATION THEORY

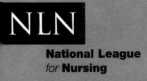

National League
for **Nursing**

THE NLN JEFFRIES SIMULATION THEORY

Edited by:

Pamela R. Jeffries, PhD, RN, FAAN, ANEF

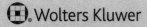

Wolters Kluwer

Philadelphia · Baltimore · New York · London
Buenos Aires · Hong Kong · Sydney · Tokyo

Acquisitions Editor: Sherry Dickinson
Product Development Editor: Dan Reilly
Production Project Manager: Marian Bellus
Design Coordinator: Stephen Druding
Illustration Coordinator: Jennifer Clements
Manufacturing Coordinator: Karin Duffield
Marketing Manager: Carolyn Fox

9 8 7 6 5 4

Printed in the United States of America

Library of Congress Cataloging-in-Publication Data

The NLN Jeffries simulation theory/edited by Pamela Jeffries; NLN.
   p. ; cm.
   National League for Nursing Jeffries simulation theory
   Includes bibliographical references.
   ISBN 978-1-934758-24-3 (alk. paper)
   I. Jeffries, Pamela R., editor, contributor. II. National League for Nursing, issuing body.
III. Title: National League for Nursing Jeffries simulation theory.
   [DNLM: 1. Education, Nursing–methods. 2. Computer Simulation. 3. Patient
Simulation. WY 18]
   RT73
   610.73071′1–dc23

                                                        2015024266

This work is provided "as is," and the publisher disclaims any and all warranties, express or implied, including any warranties as to accuracy, comprehensiveness, or currency of the content of this work.

   This work is no substitute for individual patient assessment based on health care professionals' examination of each patient and consideration of, among other things, age, weight, gender, current or prior medical conditions, medication history, laboratory data, and other factors unique to the patient. The publisher does not provide medical advice or guidance and this work is merely a reference tool. Health care professionals, and not the publisher, are solely responsible for the use of this work including all medical judgments and for any resulting diagnosis and treatments.

   Given continuous, rapid advances in medical science and health information, independent professional verification of medical diagnoses, indications, appropriate pharmaceutical selections and dosages, and treatment options should be made and health care professionals should consult a variety of sources. When prescribing medication, health care professionals are advised to consult the product information sheet (the manufacturer's package insert) accompanying each drug to verify, among other things, conditions of use, warnings and side effects and identify any changes in dosage schedule or contradictions, particularly if the medication to be administered is new, infrequently used, or has a narrow therapeutic range. To the maximum extent permitted under applicable law, no responsibility is assumed by the publisher for any injury and/or damage to persons or property, as a matter of products liability, negligence of law or otherwise, or from any reference to or use by any person of this work.

www.LWW.com   www.NLN.org

About the Editor

Dr. Pamela R. Jeffries, Dean and Professor at George Washington University (GW) School of Nursing, is nationally known for her research and work in developing simulations and online teaching and learning. Throughout the academic community, she is well regarded for her expertise in experiential learning, innovative teaching strategies, new pedagogies, and the delivery of content using technology in nursing education. Dr. Jeffries has served as principal investigator on grants with national organizations such as the National League for Nursing (NLN), has provided research leadership and mentorship on national projects with the National Council State Board of Nursing, and has served as a consultant for health care organizations, corporations, large health care organizations, and publishers, providing expertise in clinical education, simulations, and other emerging technologies. Prior to joining GW, Dr. Jeffries was Vice Provost for Digital Initiatives and professor at the School of Nursing at Johns Hopkins University, where she was previously the Associate Dean for Academic Affairs.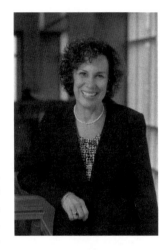

Dr. Jeffries is a Fellow of the American Academy of Nursing (FAAN), an American Nurse Educator Fellow (ANEF), and most recently, a Robert Wood Johnson Foundation Executive Nurse Fellow (ENF). She also serves as a member of the Institute of Medicine's Global Intraprofessional Education (IPE) forum and is now serving as past President of the Society in Simulation and Healthcare (SSH). She has numerous publications, is sought to deliver presentations nationally and internationally, and has just edited three books, *Simulations in Nursing Education: From Conceptualization to Evaluation*, 2nd edition, *Developing Simulation Centers Using the Consortium Model*, and her newest book, published by Lippincott and being launched at the International Meeting on Simulation in Healthcare (IMSH), called *Clinical Simulations in Nursing Education: Advanced Concepts, Trends, and Opportunities*.

She has received federal and state grants to support her research focus in nursing education and the science of innovation and learning. Jeffries was recently inducted into the prestigious Sigma Theta Tau Research Hall of Fame, and is the recipient of several teaching and research awards from the Midwest Nursing Research Society, the International Nursing Association of Clinical Simulations and Learning (INACSL), and teaching awards from the NLN and Sigma Theta Tau International. She most recently received the American Association of Colleges of Nursing (AACN) and Scholarship of Teaching and Learning Excellence Award.

About the Contributors

Katie Anne Adamson, PhD, RN, earned her Bachelor of Science in Nursing from the University of Washington Seattle. After serving as a US Navy Nurse Corps Officer, she earned her Master of Nursing from the University of Washington Bothell and PhD from Washington State University. She is a 2014–2017 Robert Wood Johnson Foundation (RWJF) Nurse Faculty Scholar. Dr. Adamson's primary areas of research include assessing the reliability and validity of instruments used to evaluate simulation participant performance and comparing learning outcomes between simulation modalities. Her RWJF-funded research compares learning outcomes between manikin-based and virtual, computer-based simulation activities. Dr. Adamson is an Assistant Professor at the University of Washington Tacoma, where she teaches in the Bachelor of Science and Master of Nursing, Bachelor of Arts in Healthcare Leadership, and Doctorate of Education Programs.

Carol Fowler Durham, EdD, RN, FAAN, ANEF is Professor and Director, Education-Innovation-Simulation Learning Environment (EISLE) at the University of North Carolina at Chapel Hill School of Nursing. Dr. Durham seamlessly integrates excellence in teaching with long-time experience in practice and scholarship to improve the ways that faculty prepare the nursing workforce of the future. As a member of the RWJFs *Quality and Safety Education for Nurses* (QSEN) project, she developed simulation-based educational experiences that reflect cutting-edge pedagogy. Dr. Durham is a visionary leader in simulation education with expertise integrating this methodology in preparing the next generation of interprofessional practitioners. She is a fellow in the American Academy of Nursing and the National League for Nursing (NLN) Academy of Nursing Education. Dr. Durham received the 2010 Academic Achievement Award from Western Carolina University and the Alumni of the Year award from the University of North Carolina and Western Carolina University in 2008. She is President of the International Nursing Association for Clinical Simulation and Learning (INACSL).

Mary Fey, PhD, RN, CHSE is the Program Manager for the Acceleration to Practice Program, National League for Nursing, and Assistant Professor at the University of Maryland School of Nursing. She has been teaching using clinical simulation since 2006. She has developed clinical simulation programs and integrated simulation into undergraduate and graduate nursing curricula.

Dr. Fey is the coauthor of the *Standard of Best Practice for Simulation: Standard VI, The Debriefing Process*. She has completed both qualitative and quantitative studies on debriefing and regularly provides faculty development to simulation educators. Her debriefing training is from the Center for Medical Simulation in Boston, Massachusetts, where she is an adjunct faculty member.

She serves on the research committee and the Standards Advisory Board of INACSL. She also serves on the Certification Committee of the Society for Simulation in Healthcare (SSH).

Dr. Fey holds a PhD and a Post-Master's Certificate in Teaching from the University of Maryland.

Susan Gross Forneris, PhD, RN, CNE, CHSE-A is the current NLN Excelsior Scholar in Residence for Simulation. Selected for inclusion in the 2010 inaugural group of NLN Simulation Leaders, she has been working in the field of clinical simulation since 2007. Dr. Forneris's expertise is in curriculum development, with emphasis on simulation and debriefing in combination with her research on critical thinking. She served as a simulation expert for the NLN ACE.S Team (Advancing Care Excellence for Seniors) and a simulation author for the NLN ACE.Z Alzheimer's simulation scenario series. She is currently the NLN project manager in the development of simulation scenarios focused on nursing assessment and fundamentals. Dr. Forneris is actively engaged in initiating multi-site simulation research on simulation and debriefing with the MN Consortium for Nursing Education and Research. She has several publications focused on the development and use of reflective teaching strategies.

Patricia K. Ravert, PhD, RN, CNE, FAAN, **ANEF,** Dean of the College of Nursing at Brigham Young University (BYU), received her undergraduate and master's degree in nursing administration from BYU and a doctorate from the University of Utah. Dr. Ravert is a Fellow in the Academy of Nursing Education with the National League for Nursing and is a Certified Nurse Educator. Her research focus is simulation learning in nursing education, particularly high-fidelity simulation. Her scholarship trajectory includes examining simulation design, integration and implementation, and evaluation of simulation experiences. Dr. Ravert was the principal investigator for a grant funded by the NLN Foundation for Nursing Education, which served as the catalyst for the work described in this monograph.

Mary Anne Rizzolo, EdD, RN, FAAN, **ANEF** began her interest in simulation in the 1980s, when she designed and developed interactive patient case study simulations using an Apple II and a Sony Betamax video player. She then pioneered the development of interactive videodisc programs that won national and international awards. During her tenure at the National League for Nursing, she was the staff liaison for all the simulation projects: the original research project from 2003 to 2006, the Simulation Innovation Resource Center (SIRC) development project, the Advancing Care Excellence in Seniors (ACES) unfolding cases, vSim projects, and the project to explore the use of simulation for high-stakes assessment. She has delivered over 200 national and international presentations, authored articles and book chapters on the use of technology in nursing, and served on many national committees and advisory boards. She currently serves on the Society for Simulation in Healthcare's Board of Directors. Dr. Rizzolo maintains an active consulting practice that includes managing several simulation projects.

Beth Rodgers, PhD, RN, FAAN is Professor and Chair of Research and PhD Studies at the University of New Mexico, College of Nursing, Albuquerque, NM. Prior to moving to Albuquerque, Dr. Rodgers enjoyed a long career at the University of Wisconsin–Milwaukee, where she conducted research on chronic illness and taught in the areas of research methods and theory development. Dr. Rodgers is known internationally for her work on nursing knowledge, theory, and concept development, as well as for her contributions to qualitative research. She has been a prominent scholar, consultant, and educator in these areas for more than three decades. She is the author of three texts; *Concept Development in Nursing* (with Dr. Kathleen Knafl), and the more recent *Developing Nursing Knowledge*, are required reading in PhD and graduate programs around the globe. She recently published a text on concept-based teaching *Mastering Concept-Based Teaching,* that is in wide use as well.

Foreword

In 2005, the National League for Nursing and Dr. Pamela Jeffries published A Framework for Designing, Implementing, and Evaluating Simulations Used as Teaching Strategies in Nursing. Since that time, the framework has become *the* essential handbook for nurse educators involved in simulation. In this monograph, titled *The NLN Jeffries Simulation Theory*, Jeffries and her team of experienced, internationally recognized nursing educators and simulationists take the important next step of moving the framework forward to create a theory of simulation in nursing.

While conceptual frameworks are descriptive, showing relevant concepts and how they relate to each other, theories tend to be specific, explain patterns seen in practice that are supported by evidence, and situate concepts in a manner that is amenable to hypothesis testing. Theories provide a basis for informed practice—something we desperately need if simulation is to be fully integrated into nursing education.

In a time when simulation is becoming an expected part of most health professions' education programs, this monograph provides clear guidance for novices as well as experts in the use of simulation in a structured and intentional manner. The monograph describes the basis for the new theoretical model and its implications for educational research.

I have had the personal and professional privilege of working with Pam and many of the authors who have contributed to this monograph. Their insights, experience, and passion shine through their work and serve to motivate and inspire those of us committed to developing the next generation of nurses into confident and competent, self-directed, life-long learners capable of being members of high-performing, high-reliability teams. I believe that the theory of simulation presented here is destined to become a major force for innovative change in nursing education.

I'm confident you will find this monograph as useful as I do.

Mary E. (Beth) Mancini, PhD, RN, NE-BC, FAHA, FAAN, ANEF
Professor
Associate Dean and Chair, Undergraduate Nursing Programs
Baylor Professor for Healthcare Research
The University of Texas at Arlington
College of Nursing and Health Innovation
Past President, The Society for Simulation in Healthcare

Preface

Theoretical thinking is essential to developing nursing science and to our professional endeavors and activities (Meleis, 2012). Theoretical activities bring organization to what we know and help to advance and clarify the nature of the discipline of nursing. Whether it is evidence-based nursing practice or evidence-based teaching, we can enhance the state of the science in nursing through processes that nurses use in conceptualizing actions through theory-based policies and theory-driven practices.

Nurses have a long history of commitment to theory-driven activities. This is demonstrated in our language of theoretical thinking and the use of theory from other disciplines to describe nursing phenomena, practices, and interventions dealing with clients' clinical problems and teaching–learning practices and behaviors. Theories describe and define phenomena and assist in clarifying relationships with other phenomena so that a nursing action, activity, or strategy can be created based on this theoretical thinking.

This commitment to theory needs to be maintained to advance knowledge in the area of simulation. The existence of clear, well-constructed, and sound theory is essential to provide a substantive foundation for research, education, and practice (Rodgers, 2005). Researchers examine theories to determine the most useful ones to build and create knowledge. Researchers explore whether a theory can help refine and explain the phenomena studied. Clinicians evaluate theories in practice, searching for the best evidence to improve health care outcomes, or in education, to foster successful learning. The professional clinician uses theory to decide what to assess in one's clients, to determine nursing actions, and to define what interventions are best for the patient/family interaction. Some decisions are based on theory, whereas others are based on theoretical thinking, not yet to the level of organized theory, but which serve as an impetus for theory development.

The NLN Jeffries theory is one such exemplar that was developed through theoretical thinking and testing as evidenced by the work done by nurse education researchers. The nursing researchers conducted activities that contributed to the development and declaration of the NLN Jeffries Simulation Framework to a simulation mid-range theory (Durham, Cato, & Lasater, 2014; Groom, Henderson, & Sittner, 2014; Hallmark, Thomas, & Gantt, 2014; Jones, Reese, & Shelton, 2014; O'Donnell, Decker, Howard, Levett-Jones, & Miller, 2014; Ravert & McAfooes, 2014). This theory is mid-range in scope, a type of theory that is less abstract than broader (grand) theories and that addresses specific phenomena or concepts that reflect practice, that is, administrative, clinical, or teaching (Meleis, 2012; Rodgers, 2005). In the past, such works might not have been considered "theory" (Rodgers, 2005); contemporary ideas, however, discuss theory in words similar to those of Meleis (2012): "An organized, coherent, and systematic articulation of a set of statements related to significant questions in a discipline and communicated as a meaningful whole" (p. 29). This theory, the revised NLN Jeffries theory, has been developed through a highly systematic process involving rigorous research and literature review, along with the perspectives of nurses immersed in simulation activities, to create a work that can be an effective guide to implementation as well as further research. The process for the development of this theory is described in this monograph.

Why is this important? Clinical simulation is a phenomenon defined as a perceived situation, a process, a group of events, and/or a group of situations. To understand the phenomenon, nursing theory is used to identify and explain relationships among phenomena, to predict consequences, or to provide action from these activities (Meleis, 2012). Not only is nursing theory an articulation of phenomena and their relationships, but such an articulation has to be communicated to the research community and to the community of people who will use the theory to guide their practices.

The challenge to nursing education researchers now is to test and use the theory to guide research in studying the simulation phenomena and to contribute to the science of nursing education. The work does not end here; it is only a beginning. Providing a mid-range nursing theory to study the phenomena of simulations can only facilitate the exploration of best practices, outcomes, and systems change through research and development of new knowledge and practices that will be discovered.

Pamela R. Jeffries, PhD, RN, FAAN, ANEF

References

Durham, C. F., Cato, M. L., & Lasater, K. (2014, July). NLN/Jeffries Simulation Framework State of the Science Project: Participant construct. *Clinical Simulation in Nursing*, *10*(7), 363–372. http://dx.doi.org/10.1016/j.ecns.2014.04.002.

Groom, J. A., Henderson, D., & Sittner, B. J. (2014). NLN/Jeffries Simulation Framework State of the Science Project: Simulation design characteristics. *Clinical Simulation in Nursing*, *10*(7), 337–344. http://dx.doi.org/10.1016/j.ecns.2013.02.004.

Hallmark, B. F., Thomas, C. M., & Gantt, L. (2014). The Educational Practices Construct of the NLN/Jeffries Simulation Framework: State of the science. *Clinical Simulation in Nursing*, *10*(7), 345–352. http://dx.doi.org/10.1016/j.ecns.2013.04.006.

Jeffries, P. R. (2005). A framework for designing, implementing, and evaluating simulations used as teaching strategies in nursing. *Nursing Education Perspectives*, *26*(2), 96–103.

Jeffries, P. R. (Ed.). (2007). *Simulation in nursing education: From conceptualization to evaluation*. New York, NY: National League for Nursing.

Jones, A. L., Reese, C. E., & Shelton, D. P. (2014). NLN/Jeffries Simulation Framework State of the Science Project: The teacher construct. *Clinical Simulation in Nursing*, *10*(7), 353–362. http://dx.doi.org/10.1016/j.ecns.2013.10.008.

Meleis, A. I. (2012). *Theoretical nursing: development and progress*. Philadelphia, PA: Lippincott Williams & Wilkins.

O'Donnell, J. M., Decker, S., Howard, V., Levett-Jones, T., & Miller, C. W. (2014). NLN/Jeffries Simulation Framework State of the Science Project: Simulation Learning Outcomes. *Clinical Simulation in Nursing*, *10*(7), 373–382. http://dx.doi.org/10.1016/j.ecns.2014.06.004.

Ravert, P., & McAfooes, J. (2014) NLN/Jeffries Simulation Framework: State of the Science Summary. *Clinical Simulation in Nursing*, *10*, 335–336. http://dx.doi.org/10.1016/j.ecns.2013.06

Rodgers, B. L. (2005). *Developing nursing knowledge: Philosophical traditions and influences*. Philadelphia, PA: Lippincott Williams & Wilkins.

Contents

About the Editor v

About the Contributors vi

Foreword ix

Preface x

List of Figures and Tables xiii

CHAPTER 1 **History and Evolution of the NLN Jeffries Simulation Theory** 1
Mary Anne Rizzolo, EdD, RN, FAAN, ANEF,
Carol Fowler Durham, EdD, RN, FAAN, ANEF,
Patricia K. Ravert, PhD, RN, CNE, FAAN, ANEF,
& Pamela R. Jeffries, PhD, RN, FAAN, ANEF

CHAPTER 2 **Systematic Review of the Literature for the NLN Jeffries Simulation Framework: Discussion, Summary, and Research Findings** 9
Katie Anne Adamson, PhD, RN,
& Beth Rodgers, PhD, RN, FAAN

CHAPTER 3 **NLN Jeffries Simulation Theory: Brief Narrative Description** 39
Pamela R. Jeffries, PhD, RN, FAAN, ANEF,
Beth Rodgers, PhD, RN, FAAN,
& Katie Anne Adamson, PhD, RN

CHAPTER 4 **NLN Vision: Teaching with Simulation** 43
Susan Gross Forneris, PhD, RN, CNE, CHSE-A,
& Mary Fey, PhD, RN, CHSE

CHAPTER 5 **Future Research and Next Steps** 51
Pamela R. Jeffries, PhD, RN, FAAN, ANEF,
Katie Anne Adamson, PhD, RN,
& Beth Rodgers, PhD, RN, FAAN

List of Figures and Tables

LIST OF FIGURES

Figure 1.1   First Iteration of The NLN Jeffries Simulation Framework   2

Figure 1.2   Second Iteration of The NLN Jeffries Simulation Framework   3

Figure 1.3   Third Iteration of The NLN Jeffries Simulation Framework   3

Figure 1.4   Fourth Iteration of The NLN Jeffries Simulation
              Framework   5

Figure 3.1   Diagram of NLN Jeffries Simulation Theory   40

LIST OF TABLES

Table 2.1   Educational Practices Components of the NLN Jeffries
              Simulation Framework   18

Table 2.2   Current Variables Listed for the Simulation Design
              Characteristics Component   23

Table 2.3   Additional Components to Support the Participant Variable   23

Table 2.4   Additional Variables Used to Describe the Facilitator   26

Table 2.5   Additional Outcome Variables Supported by the Literature   27

History and Evolution of the NLN Jeffries Simulation Theory

Mary Anne Rizzolo, EdD, RN, FAAN, ANEF
Carol Fowler Durham, EdD, RN, FAAN, ANEF
Patricia K. Ravert, PhD, RN, CNE, FAAN, ANEF
Pamela R. Jeffries, PhD, RN, FAAN, ANEF

THE BEGINNINGS

In February of 2003, Laerdal Medical Corporation (Laerdal) provided funding to the National League for Nursing (NLN) to support a national, multi-site, multi-method project to develop and test models using simulation to promote student learning in nursing. The NLN issued a nationwide call for a project director and schools that wished to be considered as project sites. Fourteen applications were received for the project director position; Pamela Jeffries was the unanimous choice. There were 175 applications from schools of nursing, and eight project sites were selected.

A kickoff meeting took place on June 23 and 24, 2003 at Laerdal Headquarters in Gatesville, Texas, attended by the project director, all project coordinators, and staff members from the NLN and Laerdal. In preparation for the meeting, everyone was asked to do a literature search and bring any articles that could be of use on the project to the meeting. Since simulation as we know it today was in its infancy in 2003, few articles were found. Even a review of journals targeted to medicine and the military that discussed related topics like role playing and use of video and CD ROMs yielded limited useful information. Few were research based, and most of the articles provided only anecdotal data.

Since no theoretical framework for simulation existed at that time, much of the meeting was spent discussing this topic. The project director provided the project coordinators with a review of the literature on constructivist, sociocultural, and learner-centered theories that had the potential to guide the development of a theoretical framework based on a collaborative technology model. Next, small groups worked on exploring various constructs related to the theories and developed questions that could guide the development of instruments to measure the constructs.

Following the June meeting, the project director devoted her time to developing the framework to design, implement, and evaluate the use of simulations in nursing education. The first image of what was originally called the "Simulation Model" can be

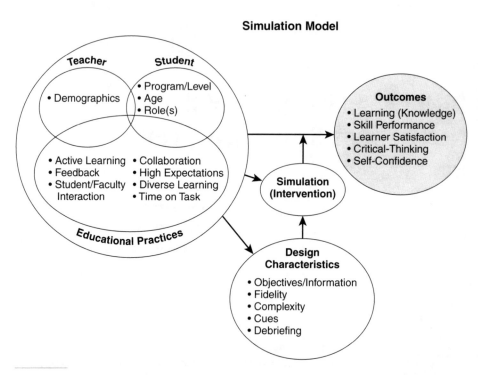

FIGURE 1.1 First Iteration of The NLN Jeffries Simulation Framework. (Reprinted with permission from Jeffries, P. R., and Rizzolo, M. A. [unpublished report, 2006]. Designing and Implementing Models for the Innovative Use of Simulation to Teach Nursing Care of Ill Adults and Children: A National, Multi-Site, Multi-Method Study.)

seen in Figure 1.1. Jeffries's article (2005), describing the framework and each of its components, appeared with a modification of the original model (Figure 1.2); a third variation appeared in Jeffries's book (2007), labeled "The Nursing Education Simulation Framework" (Figure 1.3).

INACSL TEAM EXAMINES STATE OF THE SCIENCE

In the summer of 2011, the International Nursing Association for Clinical Simulation and Learning (INACSL), in consultation with Dr. Pamela Jeffries, convened nursing simulation educators and researchers to examine the state of the science regarding simulation and the application of the Nursing Education Simulation Framework. With partial funding from an NLN Research Grant, the 21 individuals who volunteered for this project were divided into five teams, each assigned to address a different construct of the model: student, teacher, educational practices, simulation design characteristics, and outcomes. Each construct team was asked to examine the literature in light of the following questions:

1. "How is the concept defined in the literature to date?

2. What is the state of the science (what evidence is available) surrounding the assigned framework constructs to date?

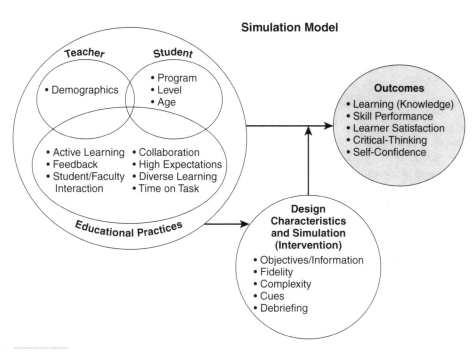

FIGURE 1.2 Second Iteration of The NLN Jeffries Simulation Framework. (Reprinted with permission from Jeffries, P.R. (2005). A framework for designing, implementing, and evaluating simulations used as teaching strategies in nursing. *Nursing Education Perspectives*, *26*(2): 96–103.)

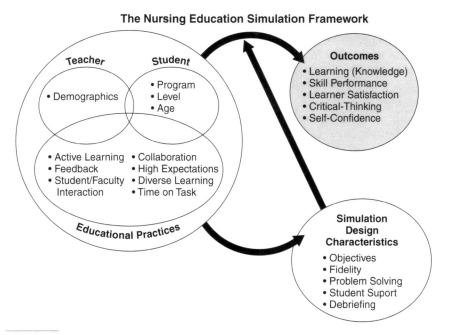

FIGURE 1.3 Third Iteration of The NLN Jeffries Simulation Framework. (Reprinted with permission from Jeffries, P. R. (Ed.). (2007). *Simulation in nursing education: From conceptualization to evaluation*. New York: National League for Nursing, p. 23.)

3. What are the major knowledge gaps and research opportunities in these areas?

4. What are the important future directions for research surrounding the concepts in the framework?" (Ravert & McAfooes, 2014, p. 335)

Hallmark, Thomas, and Gantt (2014) focused on the construct *educational practices,* and discovered that *high expectations* was seldom found in the literature. They also discovered that debriefing and feedback were different concepts in the literature, but the terms were often used interchangeably. Faculty–student interaction was supported as an important educational practice affecting confidence and retention.

Jones, Reese, and Shelton (2014) discovered that the construct *teacher* was often not defined in the simulation literature. They found that *facilitator* was more consistently used in simulation educational practices and recommended that the term *facilitator* replace the word *teacher.* They noted a lack of reliability and validity for the NLN Jeffries Simulation Framework in the literature.

Durham, Cato, and Lasater (2014) examined the construct *student* and determined that the word *participant* allowed for inclusion of the myriad of roles required in a simulation. Additionally, the review of the literature expanded the list of elements in the original framework from "program, level, and age" to "role/responsibilities, attributes, values, and demographics," providing more comprehensive descriptors of those who participate in simulation.

Groom, Henderson, and Sittner (2014) found that the construct *simulation design characteristics* was "a fundamental guiding foundation for creation, execution, and evaluation of simulation scenarios" (p. 343). They found that the simulation design characteristics—objectives, fidelity, problem solving, student support, and debriefing—were discussed in the literature but did not have strong supporting evidence.

O'Donnell, Decker, Howard, Levett-Jones, and Miller (2014) reviewed the literature for the construct *outcomes* and found that the descriptors learning (knowledge), skill performance, learner satisfaction, critical thinking, and self-confidence were widely discussed in the simulation literature but felt that key outcomes around teamwork, communication, roles, and responsibilities should also be included in outcome measurements. They also noted that "learning outcomes creates a provocative relationship between learner, simulator, educator and environment" (p. 374).

The teams involved in this initial effort to examine the Nursing Education Simulation Framework, later known as the NLN Jeffries Simulation Framework, were plagued by uncertainty about whether they had reached saturation in their search of the literature due to lack of standard terms (Ravert & McAfooes, 2014). Overall, the group found only a few empirical studies and noted variance in the strength of the available evidence to support the constructs. However, the reviews of the literature were instrumental in identifying challenges in the use of the model and uncovered such issues as lack of clarity about the name of the model and how to reference it, as well as inconsistent terminology for the constructs. Two of the research teams identified the need to broaden the names of the constructs from *teacher* to *facilitator* and from *student* to *participant.* These revised construct names were adopted by the NLN and Jeffries for the next iteration of the model (Jeffries, 2012) (Figure 1.4).

Preliminary findings were presented by the team members at the 11th Annual INACSL conference in June 2012. Manuscripts presenting the evidence for all five constructs

The NLN Jeffries Simulation Framework

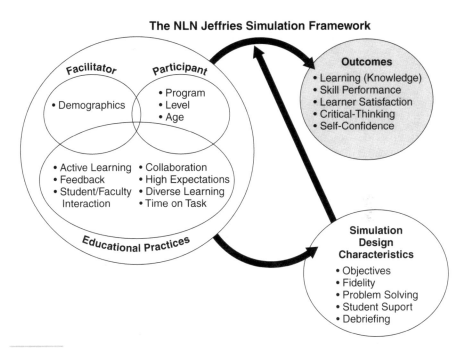

FIGURE 1.4 Fourth Iteration of The NLN Jeffries Simulation Framework. Reprinted with permission from Jeffries, P. R. (Ed.). (2012). *Simulation in nursing education: From conceptualization to evaluation.* (2nd ed.). New York: National League for Nursing, p. 37.)

were published July 2014 in *Clinical Simulation in Nursing,* providing additional information about the state of simulation, evidence for the constructs, and use of the Nursing Education Simulation Framework. There was consensus across the five research teams regarding the need for further research using the NLN Jeffries Simulation Framework to determine the impact of simulation as a modality for education and research. A published critique of the framework (LaFond & Vincent, 2013) came to similar conclusions, stating that the Framework offered promise and recommended continued research to empirically support the definitions of concepts and associated variables.

MOVEMENT TOWARD A THEORY

In October of 2012, the NLN received funding from Laerdal to underwrite some of the costs to continue this important work. An internationally known expert in theory development, Beth Rodgers, PhD, RN, FAAN, was recruited to examine the literature reviews provided by the INACSL teams and evaluate the potential for moving the NLN Jeffries Simulation Framework from a framework to a theory. A member of each of the original INACSL teams along with INACSL leaders were invited to participate in this work. Dr. Rodgers held conference calls with team members and requested that they identify significant issues or questions related to the construct that they had previously researched and conduct an initial literature review to determine the availability of research/quality evidence related to those questions. This work was to provide a basis for discussion at a think tank scheduled for June 2013, and to determine the feasibility of constructing an evidence-based foundation for testing and further development of the Framework.

The think tank was held on June 11 and 12, 2013 at the Paris Hotel in Las Vegas. Dr. Rodgers presented information on the theory development process. Over the two-day period, the group focused on identifying goals for the Framework, and discussed each concept/construct in the Framework with regard to its clarity, usefulness, and need for further development. The discussion reaffirmed the importance of the NLN Jeffries Simulation Framework and the appropriateness of its components and content.

Dr. Rodgers felt that the NLN Jeffries Simulation Framework could have been called a descriptive theory from the beginning, but recommended that in order to provide a solid theoretical foundation for quality simulation experiences, there is a need to further delineate and clarify each constituent concept or construct in the Framework and to clarify the nature of relationships among the components. This would allow for more testing and can, over time, raise the theory to an explanatory and predictive level. As a next step, she recommended the completion of a comprehensive literature review with high-quality evidence tables, focused on completed rigorous research. The intended outcome of such a thorough process would be a comprehensive review of existing research. It would not only clarify the concepts/constructs in the Framework and the relationships among the various components, but would also reveal gaps in the literature and, consequently, clear directions for further research.

In August of 2014, Dr. Katie Adamson was contracted to complete a systematic review of the literature related to the use of the NLN Jeffries Simulation Framework, working closely with and following the guidelines outlined by Dr. Rodgers. The outcomes of Dr. Adamson's work and the evolution of the NLN Jeffries Theory of Simulation are revealed in the chapters that follow.

References

Durham, C. F., Cato, M. L., & Lasater, K. (2014, July). NLN/Jeffries Simulation Framework State of the Science Project: Participant construct. *Clinical Simulation in Nursing, 10*(7), 363–372. http://dx.doi.org/10.1016/j.ecns.2014.04.002.

Groom, J. A., Henderson, D., & Sittner, B. J. (2014, July). NLN/Jeffries Simulation Framework State of the Science Project: Simulation Design Characteristics. *Clinical Simulation in Nursing, 10*(7), 337–344. http://dx.doi.org/10.1016/j.ecns.2013.02.004.

Hallmark, B. F., Thomas, C. M., & Gantt, L. (2014, July). The Educational Practices Construct of the NLN/Jeffries Simulation Framework: State of the Science. *Clinical Simulation in Nursing, 10*(7), 345–352. http://dx.doi.org/10.1016/j.ecns.2013.04.006.

Jeffries, P. R. (2005). A framework for designing, implementing, and evaluating simulations used as teaching strategies in nursing. *Nursing Education Perspectives, 26*(2), 96–103.

Jeffries, P. R. (Ed.). (2007). *Simulation in nursing education: From conceptualization to evaluation.* New York: National League for Nursing.

Jeffries, P. R. (Ed.). (2012). *Simulation in nursing education: From conceptualization to evaluation* (2nd ed.). New York, NY: National League for Nursing.

Jones, A. L., Reese, C. E., & Shelton, D. P. (2014, July). NLN/Jeffries Simulation Framework State of the Science Project: The teacher construct. *Clinical Simulation in Nursing, 10*(7), 353–362. http://dx.doi.org/10.1016/j.ecns.2013.10.008.

LaFond, C. M., & Vincent, C. V. H. (2013). A critique of the National League for Nursing/Jeffries Simulation Framework. *Journal of Advanced Nursing, 69*(2), 465–480.

O'Donnell, J. M., Decker, S., Howard, V., Levett-Jones, T., & Miller, C. W. (2014, July). NLN/Jeffries Simulation Framework State of the Science Project: Simulation Learning Outcomes. *Clinical Simulation in Nursing, 10*(7), 373–382. http://dx.doi.org/10.1016/j.ecns.2014.06.004.

Ravert, P., & McAfooes, J. (2014). NLN/Jeffries Simulation Framework: State of the Science Summary. *Clinical Simulation in Nursing, 10*, 335–336. http://dx.doi.org/10.1016/j.ecns.2013.06.002.

2

Systematic Review of the Literature for the NLN Jeffries Simulation Framework: Discussion, Summary, and Research Findings

Katie Anne Adamson, PhD, RN

Beth Rodgers, PhD, RN, FAAN

This systematic review of the literature uses the NLN Jeffries Simulation Framework as well as the five individual components of the NLN Jeffries Simulation Framework (facilitator, participant, educational practices, outcomes, and simulation design characteristics) to identify themes, gaps, and key issues that exist in the simulation literature. Findings from the systematic review help illuminate what is currently known about best simulation practices, what research exists to support these practices, and priorities for future research.

As noted previously, the development and refinement of theory is a vital aspect of the advancement of any discipline. Theory is developed through successive stages and can be accomplished using a variety of procedures. Conceptually focused activities can be used to clarify components; theoretical analysis can determine inconsistencies, gaps, and incongruencies with established theories; and empirical research provides evidence to support the elements and relationships among components of a theory. Theory can be tested directly or, in the early stages, existing research can provide guidance as to the order and connections among components. The process used in this latest phase of theory development built on the foundation provided by the initial NLN Jeffries framework (Jeffries, 2012). When the work reported in this monograph was started, the framework actually was a type of theoretical entity. The distinction between framework and theory is not always useful in actual application. The initial framework provided a critical, descriptive view of simulation experiences. It showed the primary components of the simulation experience, some of the key elements, an order to their appearance in the development and conduct of simulation, and some initial ideas about relationships and outcomes. These types of developments provide a crucial starting point in theory development and can be regarded as descriptive theory. It is unreasonable, if not impossible, to move forward with theory unless the core elements (variables or concepts) of a situation or phenomenon have been documented.

That level of description, however, does not provide the degree of guidance that is typically sought through theory. A theory is useful to the extent that it provides clear direction both for application and for further research. Over time, in spite of the many contributions that stemmed from that original framework, it was clear that there was a need to move the work to a higher level. This type of work represents a logical progression in the development of theory in which an existing statement of ideas gets filled in with more detail, directions and strengths of relationships begin to emerge, additional pieces are included, and the whole picture presented by the theory becomes more complete. The progression of theory development can be thought of as a map that, when zoomed out, gives some general shape and major landmarks associated with an area and, on zooming in, the details and actual connections among locations becomes more clear. In other words, more developed theories, or more formal theories, say more about how the person using the theory, whether for practice or research, can get where the person wants to go as well as revealing what will happen if particular routes are followed (or actions taken). The clear need was for theory that could help individuals accomplish those goals, revealing what to consider and what to expect along the route of designing and implementing simulation as well as what to do to bring about a desired outcome.

Using the existing framework as a starting point, and having identified some of the gaps and needs as well as confirming some of the components in the framework, the existing literature was subjected to a thorough and rigorous review to see what evidence existed, both theoretical and research based, that could be used to refine the theory. This approach was driven by a pragmatic perspective focused on the creation of theory that would provide sufficient guidance to promote the implementation of effective simulation and that also would offer a solid foundation for theory-based research. The development needs to be ongoing, and research built on a consistent theoretical foundation will accelerate the process of moving toward theory with relationships among elements and actions that are clear in both direction and magnitude. By continuing both research and implementation related to this theory, it will be possible to determine what constitute "good" simulation activities and to identify causal relationships along the lines of "if someone does X then Y is likely to occur." In some aspects, there already is solid evidence to indicate the preferred practices associated with quality simulation experiences. That level of specificity is provided wherever possible as derived from the literature review. In other aspects, this level of causal relationship is still in an early stage of development. The literature analysis discussed in the following section was used to develop the theory further through consideration of existing research and evidence. This review was guided by the goal of identifying existing research that would fill in gaps, provide needed clarification, and reveal evidence in support of simulation theory. This type of review also makes it possible to recognize gaps or emerging areas of practice that could shape the developing theory. Rigorous and systematic analysis, guided by the existing descriptive theory, provides an empirical basis for the current version of the theory as well as a rigorous synthesis reflecting the state of the science related to simulation. The procedures described in this monograph also demonstrate the critical interplay of theory and research, with each enhancing and focusing the other in an ongoing process of creating an improved foundation for both practice and research.

METHOD

Garrard's (2014) *Matrix Method for Health Sciences Literature Review* guided the process for the systematic review. This process involved 1) documenting a *Paper Trail* of database searches, 2) constructing *Matrices* for abstracting pertinent content from identified articles, and 3) using the *Matrices* as structured documents for the systematic analysis and synthesis of the literature. The analyses are organized according to the objectives stated by the project supervisor:

1. Discuss the recurring themes, gaps, and key issues.

2. Summarize what currently constitutes best practices and what current research supports.

3. Identify priority areas for which research is needed.

Paper Trail

This review focused on articles from the database Cumulative Index of Nursing and Allied Health Literature (CINAHL) Plus with full text, and the journal *Simulation in Healthcare*. Reference lists from key publications were also used to add depth about specific issues identified in the systematic review. In order to address the purposes of this systematic review, it was important to use the NLN Jeffries Simulation Framework as a guide. However, it was also important to consider literature that might go beyond the boundaries of the existing Framework. Therefore, two separate searches were necessary. The first search was guided by general search terms that corresponded with the five components of the NLN Jeffries Simulation Framework (facilitator, participant, educational practices, outcomes, and simulation design characteristics). The results from this search illuminated literature that was related to each of the components of the NLN Jeffries Simulation Framework but may or may not have specifically referred to the NLN Jeffries Simulation Framework. The second search, specifically using the terms "Framework (in title) AND National League for Nursing OR NLN OR Jeffries OR Simulation" uncovered articles that referred to the NLN Jeffries Simulation Framework.

Paper Trail for Search One

The initial search parameters were "Apply related terms, Research article, Scholarly/peer reviewed journals, and English language." The search dates were January 2000 to September 2014.

> Terms: Simulat* in title (to include terms such as simulation, simulator, etc.) AND
> Facilitat* OR Instruct* OR Teach* in abstract: 435
> Student OR Participant OR Learner in abstract: +559 new references (after deleting duplicates)
>   = 994
> Educational practice* OR Pedagog* in abstract: +2 new references (after deleting duplicates)
>   = 996
> Result* OR learn* OR skill* in abstract: +853 new references (after deleting duplicates) = 1849
> Objective* OR design OR fidelity OR problem solving OR support OR debrief*: +76 new
>   references (after deleting duplicates) = 1925 TOTAL

This search was then narrowed using the following major subject headings:

simulations	emergency care
computer simulation	resuscitation
patient simulation	teamwork
models, anatomic	communication
education, medical	cognition
clinical competence	task performance and anal...
education, nursing	user-computer interface
education, nursing, bacca...	decision making, clinical
teaching methods	emergency service
internship and residency	student performance appra...
students, nursing	physicians
education, clinical	disaster planning
students, nursing, baccal...	educational measurement
resuscitation, cardiopulm...	emergency medical technic...
student attitudes	heart arrest
computer assisted instruc...	multidisciplinary care te...
learning methods	teaching methods, clinica...
emergency medicine	learning
exercise physiology	pediatrics
outcomes of education	psychomotor performance
students, medical	airway management
education, interdisciplin...	staff development
virtual reality	

This reduced the "hit list" to 1250 references from CINAHL.

One journal that is not included in CINAHL that provided essential evidence for this systematic review was *Simulation in Healthcare*. Therefore, the same search terms from the CINAHL search described previously were used, yielding the following results. (Note: This electronic journal is only available from 2006 to the present.)

Terms: Simulat* in title (to include terms such as simulation, simulator, etc.) AND
Facilitat* OR Instruct* OR Teach* as keywords: 8
Student OR Participant OR Learner as keywords: 19
Educational practice* OR Pedagog* as keywords = 50
Result* OR learn* OR skill* as keywords = 149
Objective* OR design OR fidelity OR problem solving OR support OR debrief* as keywords
  = 19
Total from *Simulation in Healthcare*: 245
Total from CINAHL and *Simulation in Healthcare*: 1495 articles and abstracts

Next, systematic reviews within the results list were identified and read (approximately 30) to get an idea of what topics had previously been reviewed. After reviewing the abstracts and titles of the 1495 articles, and informed by the systematic reviews, each article abstract was appraised for inclusion in the final review based on this question: Is this article essential for understanding "what currently constitutes the best simulation practices?" Using this filter, an initial list of 149 articles was compiled for review.

Paper Trail for Search Two

In order to ensure that existing work related to the NLN Jeffries Simulation Framework was included in the review, additional searches in CINAHL and *Simulation in Healthcare* were conducted using the terms "Framework (in title) AND National League for Nursing OR NLN OR Jeffries OR Simulation." All of the filters applied in the first search with the exception "research article" were used in this search. This, along with subsequent snowball searches using the reference lists of resulting articles, provided an additional 38 articles directly referring to the NLN Jeffries Simulation Framework. The International Nursing Association for Clinical Simulation in Nursing (2011) Task Force on the NLN Jeffries Simulation Framework publications were included in these results. Both conference poster and *Clinical Simulation in Nursing* articles were initially included, but poster presentations that were later developed into articles were eliminated.

These two searches, the first guided by the components of the NLN Jeffries Framework and the second specifically looking for literature that directly referred to the framework, yielded a total of 187 articles. Step two of the *Health Sciences Literature Review* process is described by Garrard (2014): constructing *Matrices* for abstracting pertinent content from identified articles began after acquiring the PDFs of each of these articles (minus 5% that were inaccessible). Through this process, the list of articles numbering 153 was reduced even further (115 from the more general "search one" and 38 from the more specific "search two"). In order to limit potential bias for simply confirming the existing NLN Jeffries Simulation Framework, the reviews of these two groups of articles was kept separate for the initial stages of the systematic review.

RESULTS: ANALYSIS AND SYNTHESIS OF THE LITERATURE

The following narrative uses data extracted from the previously described searches. Initially, two matrices were compiled: 1) the matrix of articles identified using the components of the NLN Jeffries Simulation Framework (search one) and 2) the matrix of articles identified using the terms "NLN Jeffries Simulation Framework" (search two). From these matrices, a list of statements addressing each of the project objectives was compiled. This section addresses the following objectives:

1. Discuss the recurring themes, gaps, and key issues.
2. Summarize what currently constitutes the best practices and what current research supports.
3. Identify priority areas for which research is needed.

Recurring Themes, Gaps, and Key Issues

Each of the three most conspicuous themes from the literature included gaps and key issues for further discussion. Much of the literature supporting the first theme, "simulation works," implied a key issue around the need for higher-quality research designs and improved measurement practices to demonstrate the true impact of simulation. One noted gap associated with this theme was the dearth of valid and reliable instruments for measuring the outcomes and impact of simulation-based instruction. The second theme, "fidelity is important," was represented by the number of studies that focused on the impact of this singular simulation design feature. A key issue emerged from the literature around what aspects of fidelity are important and how these aspects impact various outcomes of simulation. The gap associated with the theme that "fidelity is important" is the lack of a standard, agreed-upon definition of fidelity. The third theme, "debriefing is where it's at," demonstrated that debriefing is a well-accepted best practice in simulation, but there is still a key issue surrounding the best strategies for how to structure debriefing activities. One specific gap is a lack of consensus about the use of video in debriefing activities.

Simulation "Works"

A recurring theme from this review is that simulation, when compared with other types of instruction, produces positive outcomes. High-quality systematic reviews and meta-analyses clearly demonstrate that simulation, when compared with baseline or no intervention, contributes to improved performance (Cook et al., 2011) and simulation, when compared with more traditional teaching strategies, is associated with superior outcomes (Cook et al., 2013). Evidence in support of simulation is strong and growing; the recent report supported by the National Council of State Boards of Nursing (NCSBN) suggested that simulation can effectively be used to replace up to 50% of clinical time (Hayden, Smiley, Alexander, Kardong-Edgren, & Jeffries, 2014). While it is generally agreed that simulation "works," the evidence supporting this claim varies in scope and quality.

Satisfaction and Confidence

In general, participants (Rezmer, Begaz, Treat, & Tews, 2011) and educators like simulation; intuitively, they believe that it leads to improved learning and performance (Baillie & Curzio, 2009; Leigh, 2008). Multiple studies concluded that simulation improves satisfaction and confidence (Kiat, Mei, Nagammal, & Jonnie, 2007; LaFond & Vincent, 2012; Smithburger, Kane-Gill, Ruby, & Seybert, 2012) and overall, participants enjoy simulation and request additional simulation experiences (Partin, Payne, & Slemmons, 2011). Roh and Lim (2014) found that precourse simulations were the single largest predictor of student satisfaction. One piece of evidence suggesting that this fervor may not be universal came from Paskins and Peile (2010) who identified two "camps" in relation to simulation affinity: simulation enthusiasts and simulation nonenthusiasts. Satisfaction and confidence, two items under the "Outcomes" component of the NLN Jeffries Simulation Framework, are widely considered low-level evaluation metrics; there is a need to compare outcomes from simulation with outcomes from other teaching and learning activities.

Comparative Effectiveness of Simulation

Within this review, multiple studies demonstrated that simulation produced superior learning outcomes when compared with more traditional lecture or didactic teaching strategies (Cooper et al., 2012; LeFlore et al., 2012; Tiffen, Corbridge, Shen, & Robinson, 2011). The systematic review and meta-analysis by Cook et al. (2012) confirmed these findings with the conclusion that, compared with other instructional strategies, high-tech simulation produced improved outcomes. The gap and key issue identified within this theme that "simulation works" is a need for higher-quality research designs and improved measurement practices (Yuan, Williams, Fang, 2012; Yuan, Williams, Fang, & Ye, 2012) to produce generalizable evidence about the effectiveness of simulation (McGaghie, 2008). One of the primary gaps in this area is the scarcity of valid and reliable instruments for measuring performance (Harder, 2010; Walsh, Sherlock, Ling, & Carnahan, 2012). Further, there is a need to explore additional criteria of "effectiveness," including patient outcomes related to simulation training. Kirkpatrick's (1998) levels of evaluation and translation science have been suggested as model frameworks for measuring the effectiveness of simulation.

Fidelity Is Important

The second theme identified through this review is that fidelity is important. The importance of fidelity to the success of simulation activities was underscored by the volume of data around this simulation design characteristic. Comparing levels of fidelity and defining fidelity were the focus of multiple studies.

Comparing "Levels" of Fidelity

There is mixed evidence about whether one level of fidelity (high, medium, or low) is superior to the others. Several studies found similar learning outcomes with various levels of fidelity (Beebe, 2012; Lane & Rollnick, 2007). However, Grady et al. (2008) found higher performance and more positive participant attitudes associated with high (vs. low) fidelity; Butler, Veltre, and Brady (2009) noted that learners perceived that high-fidelity simulation had a greater impact on their problem-solving abilities than low-fidelity simulations. Schwartz, Fernandez, Kouyoumjian, Jones, and Compton (2007) found that HPS had various advantages over case-based learning. Further, when comparing static manikin, high-fidelity simulation, and paper and pencil case study, static manikin and high-fidelity simulation were more effective in offering problem-solving opportunities and feedback (Jeffries & Rizzolo, 2006). High-fidelity simulation was associated with higher participant satisfaction, and paper and pencil case study was less effective in promoting self-confidence (Jeffries & Rizzolo, 2006).

In contrast, when doing a similar comparison between paper and pencil case study and high-fidelity simulation, Tosterud, Hedelin, and Hall-Lord (2013) found that the paper and pencil case study group was more satisfied than the high-fidelity simulation group.

Further, Yang, Thompson, and Bland (2012) noted that increased realism in simulation activities was associated with reduced confidence and judgment accuracy among participants. Looking at additional technological capacities such as offering computer-based simulations in 3 dimensions (3-D), Bai et al. (2012) noted that participants who were exposed to text-based (non-3-D) simulations reported similarly positive attitudes towards simulation as those in the 3-D simulation group. Looking at the fidelity issue through cost-effectiveness lenses, Lapkin and Levett-Jones (2011) found that medium fidelity was more cost-effective, though high fidelity had higher utility.

The "take-home message" from this recurring theme in the research is that it is necessary to identify the appropriate level of fidelity to meet the objectives of specific simulation activities (Blake & Scanlon, 2007). For example, Andreatta et al. (2014) found that an inexpensive fruit model provided adequate fidelity for teaching highly technical operative skills. In another study, the authors confirmed previous findings with their conclusion that transitioning from low to high fidelity resulted in increased confidence (Dancz, Sun, Moon, Chen, & Ozel, 2014, confirming findings from Maran & Galvin, 2003). In the end, as recommended by Hayden et al. (2014), an "adequate" level of fidelity is necessary as part of high-quality simulation activities in order to ensure high-quality simulation outcomes.

Defining Fidelity

While there is a great deal of literature comparing outcomes from simulation activities conducted at varying levels of fidelity, there is not a consistent, agreed-upon definition of fidelity or what variables should be taken into consideration when determining "levels" of fidelity. Paige and Morin (2013) described multiple dimensions of fidelity to include physical, psychological, and conceptual fidelity, each of which exist on a continuum from low to high. Hotchkiss, Biddle, & Fallacaro (2002) used "authenticity" as a measure of realism or fidelity while Dieckmann, Gaba, and Rall (2007) identified multiple dimensions of realism to include physical, semantical, and phenomenal realism. This gap in the literature is addressed by the International Nursing Association for Clinical Simulation and Learning (INACSL) Standards of Best Practice: Simulation Standard I: Terminology, in which "Fidelity" is looked at from a holistic point of view to include physical, psychological, and social factors in addition to group culture and dynamics (Meakim et al., 2013). A key issue is that simulation researchers have not adopted a single definition of fidelity that complicates efforts to synthesize and generalize evidence about best practices related to fidelity.

Debriefing Is Where It's At

Another theme from the literature is the high value placed on debriefing. Simulation researchers prioritized debriefing as a key component of simulation activities. They recognized its contributions to successful simulation and appropriately focus on several aspects of debriefing, including whether or not video enhances or detracts from the simulation debriefing process.

Debriefing Is Essential

Bremner, Aduddell, Bennett, and VanGeest (2006) identified debriefing after each simulation experience as an essential best practice when using simulation with novice nursing students. Hayden et al. (2014) qualified their landmark finding that up to 50% of clinical time may be replaced with simulation by denoting that the simulations must be of "high-quality" and accompanied by "theory-based debriefing" (p. 538). Nursing students seem to agree with the experts and identified debriefing as the most important design feature of simulation (Dobbs, Sweitzer, & Jeffries, 2006).

Clearly, debriefing is important, but what characteristics of debriefing are most effective for which desired outcomes? Deickmann et al. (2009) suggested allowing participants to do most of the talking during debriefing. Bond et al. (2006) found technical debriefing to be slightly better than cognitive debriefing among ED residents. Cheng, Eppick, Grant, Sherbino, Zendejas, and Cook (2014) found a short debriefing session to be slightly favored over a longer debriefing session. Diekmann, Molin Friis, Lippert, & Østergaard (2009) explored the interaction between facilitator and participant and found mixed responses about what an "ideal" facilitation/debriefing looked like.

Video-enhanced, Nonvideo-enhanced Debriefing

One meta-theme within the debriefing theme was about the use of video as a supplement to debriefing. Cheng et al. (2014) found negligible differences between video-enhanced and nonvideo-enhanced debriefing. Ha (2014) found that video-assisted debriefing assisted with self-reflection; however, some learners indicated that it made them feel "tired" and "humiliated," while other learners said that it boosted their self-confidence. Results from a systematic review by Levett-Jones and Lapkin (2014) about the effectiveness of debriefing affirmed that debriefing was important, but there were no significant differences with or without use of video. While this issue has been extensively investigated, the gap/question remains, "Should video-assisted debriefing be considered the 'gold standard?'"

Best Practices Supported by the Research

While none of the three primary themes that emerged from the literature review offered definitive direction about what constitutes best practices, there were several beacons of light for those seeking best practices supported by the research. Two of the key documents from this systematic review include previous systematic reviews and meta-analyses about best practices in simulation-based instruction (Cook et al., 2013; Issenberg, McGaghie, Petrusa, Gordon, and Scalese, 2005). Issenberg et al.'s (2005) Best Evidence Medical Education (BEME) Review described features and uses of high-fidelity simulations that lead to effective learning. These 10 features included *feedback, repetitive practice, curriculum integration, range of difficulty level, multiple learning strategies, capture clinical variation, controlled environment, individualized learning, defined outcomes or benchmarks,* and *simulator validity* (pp. 21–24). Each of these features was supported elsewhere in the literature. Cook et al. (2013) confirmed Issenberg et al.'s (2005) features of effective simulation and contributed additional features including *distributed practice, interactivity, mastery learning, longer time in simulation,* and *group instruction.* Of these features, only group instruction was not consistently supported by the literature as a feature of simulation that reliably improved results (p. e851). Thematic analyses of interviews with medical students about their experiences with simulation-based instruction independently (without prompting) confirmed that feedback, curricular integration,

TABLE 2.1

Educational Practices Components of the NLN Jeffries Simulation Framework

Current NLN Jeffries Simulation Framework Variables	Suggested Variables Supported by the Literature
Active learning	Interactivity
Feedback	Feedback
Student/faculty interaction	Learner-centered
Collaboration	Interactivity
High expectations	Mastery learning, defined outcomes/benchmarks
Diverse learning	Range of difficulty, multiple learning strategies, capture clinical variation, individualized learning
Time on task	Repetitive practice, deliberate practice, dose and sequence of activities

repetitive practice, multiple learning strategies, controlled environment, and simulator validity were especially valued by students (Paskins & Peile, 2010).

Educational Practices

Many of the previously described best practices supported by research address aspects of the educational practices. Table 2.1 describes the current variables listed under the educational practices component of the NLN Jeffries Simulation Framework and suggests modifications supported by the literature. Additional variables associated with educational practices that were supported by the literature include curricular integration, and use of learning theory to guide simulation research and practice.

Feedback

The literature demonstrated that feedback and expert modeling from facilitators (Abe, Kawahara, Yamashina, & Tsuboi, 2013), as well as feedback from peers (Stegmann, Pilz, Siebeck, & Fischer, 2012), improved participant learning and performance. These multiple sources of feedback and their interaction with educational practices seem to support the overlap in the NLN Jeffries Simulation Framework Venn diagram as well as the arrows indicating the impact that they have on outcomes. Halstead et al. (2011) identified a feedback-rich environment as a theme for describing quality simulation activities. Characteristics of feedback that were supported by the literature included providing immediate feedback about simulation performance (Johannesson, Olsson, Petersson, & Silén, 2010) as well as offering participants opportunities to apply what was learned through the provided feedback (Auerbach, Kessler, & Foltin, 2011). Scaringe, Chen, and Ross (2002) found that early in the learning process, both qualitative and quantitative feedback are effective, but quantitative feedback was more effective later in the learning process.

Hallmark, Thomas, and Gantt (2014) suggested that there was a need to differentiate between feedback and debriefing.

CUING AS A FORM OF FEEDBACK

Paige and Morin (2013) concluded that there are two types of cues: *conceptual cues* that help the participant achieve the instructional objectives of the simulation and *reality cues* that help the participant navigate or clarify any gaps in the fidelity of the simulation. In order to enhance the conceptual validity of a simulation, feedback in the form of cuing should be intentional, related to the objectives of the simulation, and practiced prior to the implementation of the simulation (Paige & Morin, 2013). Cues may be delivered in a variety of ways. For example, the simulation manikin or other equipment may be programmed to display a response such as an increased heart rate that the simulation participant can palpate on the manikin, or the response may be visualized on the monitor. Similarly, the simulated patient, other role actors, or the facilitator may offer feedback in the form of cues. Binder et al. (2014) found that both verbal and equipment-generated feedback was effective. Garrett, MacPhee, and Jackson (2010) indicated that participants valued timely cues such as patient status changes.

Learner-Centered Practices

The literature did not explicitly address student/faculty interaction or collaboration. However, there was evidence suggesting that simulation activities should be learner centered. Nicholson (2012) concluded that simulations should be designed to meet learners' needs, promote learner engagement, and consider environmental safety. Learner/teacher collaboration, such as formative assessment and participant involvement in planning of simulation activities, helped meet participants' specific learning needs (Elfrink, Nininger, Rohig, & Lee, 2009). Bremner et al. (2006) and Montan et al. (2014) found that collaboration between facilitators and participants in the planning, implementation, and evaluation of simulation activities was helpful.

Time on Task Reframed as Dose–Response

Numerous studies confirmed a dose–response effect with simulation exposure and learning outcomes. Beebe (2012) found that as the number of hours of clinical simulation increased, critical thinking and knowledge scores increased. Both Kennedy, Maldonado, and Cook (2013) and McGaghie, Issenberg, Petrusa, and Scalese (2006) confirmed that longer simulation exposure correlated with improved learning outcomes. Other researchers confirmed that repeated exposure to clinical scenarios through simulation was especially effective (Abe et al., 2013; Auerbach et al., 2011; Johannesson et al., 2010). Finally, while most of the literature supporting repetitive practice and "increased" exposure to simulation did not quantify what an appropriate amount of simulation should be, Childs and Sepples (2006) suggested that a simulation lasting 25 minutes with a 10-minute session for debriefing was too short.

Mastery Learning with Deliberate Practice

A related aspect of educational practices that was supported by the literature included the use of mastery learning with deliberate practice. In short, mastery learning refers to competency-based educational strategies with standardized outcomes and deliberate practice refers to repetitive rehearsal to develop and maintain knowledge, skill, or ability. Barsuk, McGaghie, Cohen, O'Leary, and Wayne (2009) found that students trained with simulation that included mastery learning and deliberate practice showed improved patient care over students who were trained with traditional methods. Further supporting deliberate practice, McGaghie et al. (2006) found a strong dose–response relationship between the numbers of hours participants spent practicing in simulation and improved learning outcomes. The specific components of mastery learning and deliberate practice cited by McGaghie et al. (2006) included intense, repetitive performance of intended cognitive or psychomotor skills in a focused domain and rigorous skill assessment that provided learners with specific feedback that yields increasingly better skills performance in a controlled setting.

Sequencing

If more is better, it is important to consider how to best sequence elements within simulation activities and how to sequence simulation activities with other learning activities. Evidence supports creating each simulation activity with a clear beginning and end (Dieckmann et al., 2007) and sequencing of elements within a simulation to progress from briefing to simulation to debriefing (Cant & Cooper, 2009). Meyer, Connors, Hou, and Gajewski (2011) reported that students who participated in simulation before their actual patient-care experiences demonstrated improved clinical performance. This was confirmed and expanded on by Schlairet and Fenster (2012), who compared different dosing and sequencing schemes for simulation and clinical, and found that an "interleaved" scheme in which simulation preceded clinical was most effective. Further, as previously mentioned, Dancz et al. (2014) found that sequencing simulation experiences so that they transition from lower to higher fidelity increased participant confidence. On a final note about sequencing, it was noted that if simulation is used for assessment, it must first be used for learning (Botezatu, Hult, Tessma, & Fors, 2010).

Additional Educational Practices

Educational practices discussed in the literature that are not covered by the NLN Jeffries Simulation Framework included curricular integration and use of theory.

CURRICULAR INTEGRATION

Curricular integration was an educational practice described in the literature that is not reflected in the NLN Jeffries Simulation Framework. Simulation scenarios should be standardized and integrated into the curriculum (Cant & Cooper, 2009; Lucisano & Talbot, 2012). This allows for thoughtful sequencing and use of repetition to enforce concepts (Brim, Venkatan, Gordon, & Alexander, 2010). Further, simulation is not an add-on. It should be thoughtfully used to augment learning and is especially useful for providing experiences that are rare in clinical practice (Cooper et al., 2012). Foster, Sheriff, and Cheney (2008) found that grouping simulation scenarios with other educational activities such as lectures was more effective than simulations alone. Similarly, Deering et al. (2006) used simulation to enforce previous learning, and found that this practice improved participants' comfort with skills.

USE OF THEORY

Kaakinen and Arwood (2009) found that theory was a missing component in most simulation research and Rourke, Schmidt, and Garga (2010) agreed that most simulation literature does not adequately address theoretical underpinnings. Wong et al. (2008) suggested using problem-based learning to support an ideal simulation learning environment.

Diverse Learning

Fountain and Alfred (2009) indicated that various components of simulation appealed to diverse learning styles. For example, more social learners benefited from the interactive aspects of simulation while more solitary learners benefited from observation and reflection. Johannesson et al. (2010) found that variation in patient cases enhanced "fun" and the "joy of learning" in simulation.

Simulation Design Characteristics

Similar to the findings of Groom, Henderson, and Sittner (2014) and Kardong-Edgren, Starkweather, and Ward (2008), my review of the literature largely confirmed the simulation design characteristics construct within the NLN Jeffries Simulation Framework, but provided limited best practices. One source of guidance about designing evidence-based scenarios came from Waxman (2010). Drawing from her review of the literature and experience with the Bay Area Simulation Collaborative, Waxman (2010) recommended the use of evidence-based guidelines for simulation scenario development including: 1) ensuring that the learning objectives are defined; 2) identifying the level of fidelity; 3) defining the level of complexity; 4) using evidence-based references; 5) incorporating instructor prompts and cues; and 6) allowing adequate time for debriefing or guide reflection (Table 2.2).

Objectives

There was overwhelming confirmation in the literature that simulation activities should be goal directed (Brydges, Mallette, Pollex, Carnahan, & Dubrowski, 2012; Dieckmann et al., 2007; Garrett et al., 2010; Rosen, Hunt, Pronovost, Federowicz, & Weaver, 2012). Smith and Roehrs (2009) found that clear objectives geared at an appropriately challenging goal were correlated with increased satisfaction and confidence. One of the advantages of simulation is that it effectively allows adult learners to address their self-directed learning goals (Kaakinen & Arwood, 2009). The literature was also clear that learning objectives should guide the selection of simulation modality. For example, Kennedy et al. (2013) showed that virtual simulation offered advantages over other types of simulation because it allowed learners to engage in activities with increasing complexity or difficulty, and provided automated feedback and repetition.

Fidelity

Fidelity emerged as a key theme from the overall review of the literature, therefore is primarily covered in the Recurring Themes, Gaps, and Key Issues section of this chapter. However, a few aspects of fidelity specifically addressing simulation design are discussed here. Overall, the fidelity of the physical environment was considered an important aspect of simulation design, and appropriate participant orientation to the environment supported success (Cant & Cooper, 2009; DeCarlo, Collingridge, Grant, & Ventre, 2008; Kiat et al., 2007). Fidelity, as discussed earlier, should be considered a quality beyond the sophistication of the manikin (Howard, Ross, Mitchell, & Nelson, 2010). Learners may also support the fidelity of simulation activities by wearing appropriate attire, demonstrating professionalism (Hope, Garside, & Prescott, 2011), and participating appropriately as simulated patients and family members (Nicholson, 2012).

Referring to the design of the simulation, Dancz et al. (2014) confirmed previous findings of Maran and Galvin (2003) with their conclusion that transitioning from low to high fidelity resulted in increased confidence. These transitions should be deliberate and should not take place within a given simulation experience. Deckers (2011) indicated that within a given simulation experience, consistency in fidelity improved learning and that lapses or interruptions within the experience should be avoided. An exemplar for using the appropriate transitions in fidelity for the purposes of specific simulation activities was provided by Matos and Raemer (2013), who used high-fidelity manikins to simulate an adverse event and a standardized patient encounter to practice communication skills associated with error disclosure after the adverse event.

Filming

While most of the literature about filming refers to the simulation design characteristic of debriefing, there was substantial documentation in the literature about the effects of filming and "being watched" as simulation design characteristics. DeCarlo et al. (2008) indicated that being filmed was a barrier to nurses' participation in simulation while Kelly, Hager, and Gallagher (2014) found that filming ranked low in terms of what "mattered" most in simulation activities. Parker, Corey, and Myrick (2012) found that observation was considered a "threat" by participants and that disbelief (not "buying in" to the scenario) was used as a defense mechanism to counteract the threat. In the end, Trokan-Mathison (2013) indicated that being watched in simulation was less stressful than clinical.

Table 2.2 describes the current variables listed under the simulation design characteristics component of the NLN Jeffries Simulation Framework and suggested modifications supported by the literature.

Participant

The literature recognized that the contributions of simulation participants are much more complex than the three variables identified in the NLN Jeffries Simulation Framework (program, level, age). Table 2.3 identifies additional variables that should be considered for addition to the framework.

Researchers identified multiple participant-related variables that influence performance including age, gender, readiness to learn, personal goals, preparedness, tolerance for ambiguity, self-confidence, learning style, cognitive load, and level of anxiety (Beischel, 2013; Brydges et al., 2012; Diez et al., 2013; Fenske, Harris, Aebersold, & Hartman, 2013; Fountain & Alfred, 2009; Fraser et al., 2012; Ironside, Jeffries, & Martin, 2009; Jeffries, 2005; Jeffries & Rogers, 2012; Shinnick, Woo, & Evangelista, 2012). As previously mentioned, various

TABLE 2.2

Current Variables Listed for the Simulation Design Characteristics Component

Current NLN Jeffries Simulation Framework Variables	Suggested Variables Supported by the Literature
Objectives	Goals and objectives, defined outcomes or benchmarks (multiple)
Fidelity	Multiple dimensions of realism (Dieckmann et al. 2007) Multiple dimensions of fidelity (Paige & Morin, 2013) Authenticity (Hotchkiss et al., 2002)
Problem solving	Scenario complexity (Guhde, 2011)
Student support	—
Debriefing	Briefing, simulation, debriefing (Cant & Cooper, 2009)

components of the simulation experience appeal to and are effective for individuals with diverse learning preferences (Fountain & Alfred, 2009; Shinnick et al., 2012). Counterintuitively, Beischel (2013) found that a strong hand-on learning style was negatively correlated with learning in simulation. Fraser et al. (2012) found that increased participant cognitive load was associated with poorer learning outcomes. Learners who set personal goals for simulation activities demonstrated better performance in procedural skills (Brydges et al., 2012). Beischel (2013) found that participants who were more "ready to

TABLE 2.3

Additional Components to Support the Participant Variable

Current NLN Jeffries Simulation Framework Variables	Suggested Variables Supported by the Literature
Program	Age (Fenske et al., 2013)
Level	Gender (Diez et al., 2013)
Age	Readiness to learn (Beischel, 2013)
	Personal goals (Brydges et al. 2012; Kaakinen & Arwood, 2009)
	Preparedness for simulation (Beischel, 2013)
	Tolerance for ambiguity (Ironside et al. 2009)
	Self-confidence (Jeffries, 2005; Jeffries & Rogers, 2012)
	Learning style (Beischel, 2013; Fountain & Alfred, 2009; Shinnick et al., 2012)
	Cognitive load (Fraser et al., 2012; Parker et al., 2012)
	Level of anxiety (Beischel, 2013; Leblanc et al., 2012)

learn" were less anxious while those who spent more than one hour preparing for simulation activities were more anxious.

Participant Factors Under the Participants' Control

Many participant-associated factors that influenced the simulation experience are influenced by the facilitator, educational practices, and simulation design characteristics, but are largely within the control of the participants themselves. Participants' motivations, enthusiasm, and personal feelings about simulation, as well as their willingness to suspend disbelief, affected their ability to fully immerse themselves in simulation activities (Kiat et al., 2007; Leighton & Sholl, 2009; van Soeren et al., 2011). Further, participants who wore their uniforms and displayed professionalism supported the realism of the simulation experience (Diekmann et al., 2007; Hope et al., 2011) which, in turn, improved participant engagement (van Soeren et al., 2011).

Participant Factors Under the Facilitator's Control

Some participant-associated factors that influenced the simulation experience are largely within the control of the facilitator. For this reason, they may be considered variables more closely associated with the educational practices or simulation design characteristics components of the NLN Jeffries Simulation Framework. These variables include role assignment, orientation, and group size.

ROLE ASSIGNMENT

In relationship to role assignment, Kaplan, Abraham, and Gary (2012) found that the role of the observer provided an effective form of simulation learning while Jeffries and Rizzolo (2006) found that role assignment did not affect learning outcomes, but observers rated simulation lower in the area of collaboration. Zulkosky (2012) found that viewing a prerecorded simulation was less effective than participating in a case study and lecture. Kelly et al. (2014) found that students ranked their role assignment in simulation lower than other simulation variables as a contributor to their ability to develop clinical judgment while van Soeren et al. (2011) found that participants valued being able to play the role of their own profession.

ORIENTATION

A delphi study about quality indicators for simulation demonstrated that participants should be oriented to the simulation environment (Arthur, Levett-Jones, & Kable, 2013). Bambini, Washburn, and Perkins (2009) found that participants' previous experience with simulation did not affect outcomes for novice nursing students.

GROUP SIZE

There is extensive literature about the ideal number of participants in a simulation activity. Clearly, the objectives of the simulation will largely determine the appropriate number of participants, but the following evidence may be used to inform simulation practice. Partin et al. (2011) found that students expressed dissatisfaction when there were more than six students in a group and suggested that the faculty-to-manikin ratio should be one-to-one. Rezmer et al. (2011) found that group size (up to four) had no effect. This would lead one to conclude that best practice might look like four to six participants with one facilitator and one manikin. Some conflicting evidence comes from Cook et al. (2013), who found that group training had small negative effects, and Shanks, Brydges, den Brok, Nair, and Hatala (2013) who found that learning in pairs was more effective than individual learning. Hope et al. (2011) found that small groups were preferred over larger groups.

Participant/Facilitator Interaction

One notable dynamic of the NLN Jeffries Simulation Framework is the interaction between facilitator and participant. The literature clearly acknowledged one area where the two roles overlap. This was in the area of self-directed and peer-lead simulation activities. Brydges, Nair, Ma, Shanks, and Hatala (2012) found that self-directed learning in simulation lead to improved skill retention and higher correlations between confidence and competence. In further support of self-directed learning, Boet et al. (2011) found no difference in anesthesia residents' performance when they completed self- or instructor-led debriefing. Similarly, Karnath, Das Carlo, and Holden (2004) found similar learning outcomes with independent or faculty-led computer simulations. In contrast, LeFlore and Anderson (2009) found that instructor-led learning was more effective than self-directed learning in simulation and Marmol et al. (2012) found that tutor-assisted learning was more effective than self-directed learning in simulation.

Facilitator

Like with the participant construct, the literature recognized that the contributions of simulation facilitators are much more complex than the single variable identified in the NLN Jeffries Simulation Framework (demographics). In addition to understanding the theoretical/pedagogical underpinnings of simulation, facilitators need to be self-aware and help reduce obstacles that may threaten participants' ability to learn (Parker et al., 2012). Paige (2014) eloquently asserted that nurse educators in this role "facilitate discovery" and emotionally prepare and support students.

Facilitators should embrace a learner-center, "guide on the side" approach to facilitation (van Soeren et al., 2011). Behaviors that promote this approach include allowing participants to do most of the talking during debriefing (Dieckmann et al., 2009) and recognizing that not all "facilitation" must be led by the "facilitator." Computer-assisted facilitation in the form of voice-advisory manikins has been shown to improve hand position and compression rates in cardiopulmonary resuscitation (Diez et al., 2013). Additionally, nonfaculty RNs may assist with facilitation (Foster et al., 2008) and standardized patients (Bokken, Linssen, Scherpbier, vander Bleuten, & Rethans, 2009) and educational/technical support staff are valuable members of the facilitation team (Cant & Cooper, 2009). Further, as discussed previously in the Participant section of this chapter, participants may effectively act as facilitators.

Parsh (2010) interviewed undergraduate nursing students and simulation instructors to identify characteristics that each group thought contributed to effective simulated clinical experiences. Facilitator characteristics that students identified as important included personality, teaching ability, evaluation, nursing competence, interpersonal

TABLE 2.4

Additional Variables Used to Describe the Facilitator

Current NLN Jeffries Simulation Framework Variables	Suggested Variables Supported by the Literature
Demographics	Personality, nursing competence, interpersonal relationships, technological skills (Parsh, 2010)
	Attitude (Kawahara et al., 2013)
	Attributes, roles, responsibilities, values (Jones, Reese, & Shelton, 2014)
	Self-awareness (Parker et al., 2012)
	Teaching ability (Parker et al., 2012; Parsh, 2010)

relationships, and realism. Facilitator characteristics that simulation facilitators identified as important included evaluation, nursing competence, personality, teaching ability, technological skills, designing scenarios, and manipulating equipment. Encouragement and positive feedback from facilitators has been shown to motivate participants and improve performance (Abe et al., 2013) while facilitator preparation and training were identified by experts as important characteristics that facilitators bring to the simulation (Arthur et al., 2013). Finally, the INACSL Standard V: Facilitator identifies demographics, attributes, roles and responsibilities, and values as important factors describing facilitators (Jones, Reese, & Shelton, 2014). Table 2.4 describes variables in the current NLN Jeffries Simulation Framework and suggested variables supported by the literature.

Outcomes

The literature confirmed the importance of the five variables in the outcomes component of the NLN Jeffries Simulation Framework. However, it made a strong case for expanding the scope to include longer-term educational outcomes as well as the impact indicators from simulation such as patient care outcomes (Brim et al., 2010). Large amounts of evidence exist about how simulation contributes to knowledge acquisition, satisfaction, and clinical skill attainment. O'Donnell, Decker, Howard, Levette-Jones, and Miller (2014) indicated that there was less evidence demonstrating that simulation contributes to self-confidence and self-efficacy, but this finding is in conflict with other sources (LaFond & Vincent, 2012; Norman, 2012) and my own experience. A review of the literature by Rosen et al. (2012) found that a larger percentage of articles focused on learner reactions to simulation (31%) than on other outcomes such as learning (3%), behavior change (21%), and outcomes (17%).

As indicated at the beginning of this chapter, simulation "works." In addition to the evidence already provided, the literature demonstrated several novel examples of outcomes from simulation. Yuan et al. (2012) and Yuan et al. (2012) found mixed contributions of simulation to confidence and competence; simulation clearly improved scores on knowledge and skills assessments but not on objective structured clinical examination (OSCE) performance. Koskinen, Abdelhamid, & Likitalo (2008) noted that simulation exercises increase cultural and self-awareness. Simulation performance outcome measures provided valid assessments of empathy (Berg, Majdan, Berg, Veloski, & Hojat, 2011) and assessments of simulation outcomes effectively approximated critical thinking metrics (Fero et al., 2010).

One looming question in the area of outcomes remains: Do gains realized in the simulation environment transfer to the clinical environment to impact patient care? While McGaghie, Issenberg, Barsuk, and Wayne (2014) found that the "downstream" effects of simulation have been demonstrated, Finan et al. (2012) produced evidence suggesting that participants who demonstrated improved performance in the simulated environment did not necessarily perform better during actual patient care. Using Kirkpatrick's (1998) levels of evaluation—reaction, learning, behavior, and results—or translational science terminology, we can interpret this evidence to mean that, while simulation-based training can and does affect patient care, we cannot assume that upstream participant reactions and learning necessarily translate into downstream behaviors and results.

The take-away message from this is that we cannot depend on research documenting outcomes such as learning, skill performance in the simulation lab, learner satisfaction, critical thinking, and self-confidence as adequate evidence for the effectiveness of simulation. Like Fisher and King (2013) suggested, we must pursue higher levels of outcome evaluation that will inform us about whether or not learners are ready for practice. Additionally, we need to complete longitudinal research looking at multiple levels of evaluation: reaction, learning, behavior, and results/impact of simulation (Kirkpatrick, 1998).

Recommendations from the literature regarding effective outcome measurements included triangulating simulation evaluation data with other assessments to assess validity (Mudumbai, Gaba, Boulet, Howard, & Davies, 2012; Wright et al., 2013). Table 2.5 summarizes variables in the current NLN Jeffries Simulation Framework and suggests additional variables supported by the literature.

In conclusion, this narrative has used data extracted from two matrices: the matrix of articles identified using the components of the NLN Jeffries Simulation Framework (search one, Appendix A) and the matrix of articles identified using the terms, "NLN Jeffries Simulation Framework" (search two, Appendix B) to address the following objectives: 1) Discuss the recurring themes, gaps, and key issues; 2) summarize what currently

TABLE 2.5

Additional Outcome Variables Supported by the Literature

Current NLN Jeffries Simulation Framework Variables	Suggested Variables Supported by the Literature
Learning (knowledge)	Self-efficacy (O'Donnell et al., 2014)
Skill performance	Behavior change (Rosen et al., 2012)
Learner satisfaction	Patient outcomes (McGaghie et al., 2014; Rosen et al., 2012)
Critical thinking	Cultural and self-awareness (Koskinen et al., 2008)
Self-confidence	Attitudes and empathy (Berg et al., 2011)

constitutes best practices and what current research supports; and 3) identify priority areas for which research is needed. The findings from this systematic review of the literature largely supported the components of the NLN Jeffries Simulation Framework and suggested modifications or additions to the existing variables. In addition to the specific examples provided in the Results section, several articles from the systematic review provided general comments on the validity of the NLN Jeffries Simulation Framework in diverse settings. Reese, Jeffries, and Engum (2010) found that the NLN Jeffries Framework was applicable for interdisciplinary simulation, Wilson and Hagler (2012) supported the use of the framework in an acute care setting, and Young and Shellenbarger (2012) found it useful for nurse educator preparation. Additionally, findings from Cordeau's (2012) Grounded Theory work about high-stakes clinical simulation supported the NLN Jeffries Simulation Framework. One critique of the NLN Jeffries Simulation Framework by LaFond and Vincent (2012) identified weaknesses within the Framework and suggested that additional empirical support for the components and variables would improve its relevance. We believe this systematic review of the literature has substantively addressed this suggestion, and will contribute to the development of the Framework.

References

Abe, Y., Kawahara, C., Yamashina, A., & Tsuboi, R. (2013). Repeated scenario simulation to improve competency in critical care: A new approach for nursing education. *American Journal of Critical Care, 22*(1), 33–40. doi:10.4037/ajcc2013229

Andreatta, P., Marzano, D., Curran, D., Klotz, J., Gamble, C., & Reynolds, R. (2014). Low-hanging fruit: A clementine as a simulation model for advanced laparoscopy. *Simulation in Healthcare: The Journal of the Society for Simulation in Healthcare, 9*, 234–240. doi:10.1097/SIH.0000000000000032

Arthur, C., Levett-Jones, T., & Kable, A. (2013). Quality indicators for the design and implementation of simulation experiences: A delphi study. *Nurse Education Today, 33*(11), 1357–1361. doi:10.1016/j.nedt.2012.07.012

Auerbach, M., Kessler, D., & Foltin, J. C. (2011). Repetitive pediatric simulation resuscitation training. *Pediatric Emergency Care, 27*(1), 29–31. doi:10.1097/PEC.0b013e3182043f3b

Bai, X., Duncan, R. O., Horowitz, B. P., Graffeo, J. M., Glodstein, S. L., & Lavin, J. (2012). The added value of 3D simulations in healthcare education. *International Journal of Nursing Education, 4*(2), 67–72. Retrieved from http://search.ebscohost.com/login.aspx?direct=true&db=rzh&AN=2011793111&site=ehost-live

Baillie, L. & Curzio, J. (2009). Students' and facilitators' perceptions of simulation in practice learning. *Nurse Education in Practice, 9*(5), 297–306.

Bambini, D., Washburn, J., & Perkins, R. (2009). Outcomes of clinical simulation for novice nursing students: Communication, confidence, clinical judgment. *Nursing Education Perspectives, 30*(2), 79–82.

Barsuk, J. H., McGaghie, W. C., Cohen, E. R., O'Leary, K., & Wayne, D. B. (2009). Simulation-based mastery learning reduces complications during central venous catheter insertion in a medical intensive care unit. *Critical Care Medicine, 37*(10), 2697–2701. Retrieved from http://search.ebscohost.com/login.aspx?direct=true&db=rzh&AN=2010459626&site=ehostlive

Beebe, R. I. (2012). *Relationship between fidelity and dose of human patient simulation, critical thinking skills, and knowledge in an associate degree nursing program.* West Virginia University. Doctoral dissertation. Retrieved from UMI number 3538233.

Beischel, K. P. (2013). Variables affecting learning in a simulation experience: A mixed methods study. *Western Journal of Nursing Research, 35*(2), 226–247.

Berg, K., Majdan, J. F., Berg, D., Veloski, J., & Hojat, M. (2011). A comparison of medical students' self-reported empathy with simulated patients' assessments of the students' empathy. *Medical Teacher, 33*(5), 388–391. doi:10.3109/0142159X2010.530319

Binder, C., Schmölzer, G. M., O'Reilly, M., Schwaberger, B., Urlesberger, B., & Pichler, G. (2014). Human or monitor feedback to improve mask ventilation during simulated neonatal cardiopulmonary resuscitation. *Archives of Disease in Childhood—Fetal & Neonatal Edition, 99*(2), F120–123. doi:10.1136/archdischild-2013-304311

Blake, C., & Scanlon, E. (2007). Reconsidering simulations in science education at a distance: Features of effective use. *Journal of Computer Assisted Learning, 23*(6), 491–502. doi:10.1111/j.1365-2729.2007.00239.x

Boet, S., Bould, M. D., Bruppacher, H. R., Desjardins, F., Chandra, D. B., & Naik, V. N. (2011). Looking in the mirror: Self-debriefing versus instructor debriefing for simulated crises. *Critical Care Medicine, 39*(6), 1377–1381. doi:10.1097/CCM.0b013e31820eb8be

Bokken, L., Linssen, T., Scherpbier, A., van der Vleuten, C., & Rethans, J. (2009). Feedback by simulated patients in undergraduate medical education: A systematic review of the literature. *Medical Education, 43*(3), 202–210. doi:10.1111/j.1365-2923.2008.03268.x

Bokken, L., Van Dalen, J., Scherpbier, A., van der Vleuten, C., & Rethans, J. (2009). Lessons learned from an adolescent simulated patient educational program: Five years of experience. *Medical Teacher, 31*(7), 605–612. doi:10.1080/01421590802208891

Bond, W. F., Deitrick, L. M., Eberhardt, M., Barr, G. C., Kane, B. G., Worrilow, C. C.,... Croskerry, P. (2006). Cognitive versus technical debriefing after simulation training. *Academic Emergency Medicine, 13*(3), 276–283. Retrieved from http://search.ebscohost.com/login.aspx?direct=true&db=rzh&AN=2009231674&site=ehost-live

Botezatu, M., Hult, H., Tessma, M. K., & Fors, U. (2010). Virtual patient simulation for learning and assessment: Superior results in comparison with regular course exams. *Medical Teacher, 32*(10), 845–850. doi:10.3109/01421591003695287

Bremner, M. N., Aduddell, K., Bennett, D. N., & VanGeest, J. B. (2006). The use of human patient simulators: Best practices with novice nursing students. *Nurse Educator, 31*(4), 170–174. Retrieved from http://search.ebscohost.com/login.aspx?direct=true&db=rzh&AN=2009251311&site=ehost-live

Brewer, E. P. (2011). Successful techniques for using human patient simulation in nursing education. *Journal of Nursing Scholarship, 43*(3), 311–317. doi:10.1111/j.1547-5069.2011.01405.x

Brim, N., Venkatan, S., Gordon, J., & Alexander, E. (2010). Long-term educational impact of a simulator curriculum on medical student education in an internal medicine clerkship. *Simulation in Healthcare: The Journal of the Society for Simulation in Healthcare, 5,* 75–81. doi:10.1097/SIH.0b013e3181ca8edc

Brydges, R., Mallette, C., Pollex, H., Carnahan, H., & Dubrowski, A. (2012). Evaluating the influence of goal setting on intravenous catheterization skill acquisition and transfer in a hybrid simulation training context. *Simulation in Healthcare: The Journal of the Society for Simulation in Healthcare, 7,* 236–242. doi:10.1097/SIH.0b013e31825993f2

Brydges, R., Nair, P., Ma, I., Shanks, D., & Hatala, R. (2012). Directed self-regulated learning versus instructor-regulated learning in simulation training. *Medical Education, 46*(7), 648–656. doi:10.1111/j.1365-2923.2012.04268.x

Butler, K. W., Veltre, D. E., & Brady, D. S. (2009). Implementation of active learning pedagogy comparing low-fidelity simulation versus high-fidelity simulation in pediatric nursing education. *Clinical Simulation in Nursing, 5,* e129–e136. doi:10.1016/j.ecns.2009.03.118.

Cant, R. P., & Cooper, S. J. (2009). Simulation-based learning in nurse education: Systematic review. *Journal of Advanced Nursing, 66*(1), 3–15. doi:10.1111/j.1365-2648.2009.05240.x

Cheng, A., Eppich, W., Grant, V., Sherbino, J., Zendejas, B., & Cook, D. A. (2014). Debriefing for technology-enhanced simulation: A systematic review and meta-analysis. *Medical Education, 48*(7), 657–666. doi:10.1111/medu.12432

Childs, J. C. & Sepples, S. (2006). Clinical teaching by simulation: lessons learned from a complex patient care scenario. *Nursing Education Perspectives, 27*(3), 154–158.

Cook, D. A., Hamstra, S. J., Brydges, R., Zendejas, B., Szostek, J.,H., Wang, A. T.,... Hatala, R. (2013). Comparative effectiveness of instructional design features in simulation-based education: Systematic review and meta-analysis. *Medical Teacher, 35*(1), e844–875. doi:10.3109/01421 59X.2012.714886

Cook, D. A., Hatala, R., Brydges, R., Zendejas, B., Szostek, J. H., Wang, A. T.,... Hamstra, S. J. (2011). Technology-enhanced simulation for health professions education: A systematic review and meta-analysis. *JAMA: The Journal of the American Medical Association, 306*(9), 978–988. doi:10.1001/jama.2011.1234

Cooper, S., Cant, R., Porter, J., Bogossian, F., McKenna, L., Brady, S., & Fox-Young, S. (2012). Simulation based learning in midwifery education: A systematic review. *Women & Birth, 25*(2), 64–78. doi:10.1016/j.wombi.2011.03.004

Cordeau, M. A. (2012). Linking the transition: A substantive theory of high-stakes clinical simulation. *Advances in Nursing Science, 35*(3), E90–e102. Retrieved from http://search.ebscohost.com/login.aspx?direct=true&db=rzh&AN=2011659256&site=ehost-live

Dancz, C., Sun, V., Moon, H., Chen, J., & Ozel, B. (2014). Comparison of 2 simulation models for teaching obstetric anal sphincter repair. *Simulation in Healthcare: The Journal of the Society for Simulation in Healthcare, 9*, 325–330. doi:10.1097/SIH.0000000000000043

DeCarlo, D., Collingridge, D., Grant, C., & Ventre, K. (2008). Factors influencing nurses' attitudes toward simulation-based education. *Simulation in Healthcare: The Journal of the Society for Simulation in Healthcare, 3*, 90–96. doi:10.1097/SIH.0b013e318165819e

Deckers, C. (2011). *Designing high fidelity simulation to maximize student registered nursing decision-making ability.* Pepperdine University. Doctoral dissertation Retrieved from UMI Number 3449818.

Deering, S., Hodor, J., Wylen, M., Poggi, S., Nielsen, P., & Satin, A. (2006). Additional training with an obstetric simulator improves medical student comfort with basic procedures. *Simulation in Healthcare: The Journal of the Society for Simulation in Healthcare, 1*(1), 32–34. Retrieved from http://ovidsp.ovid.com/ovidweb.cgi?T=JS&PAGE=reference&D=ovfth&NEWS=N&AN=01266021-200600110-00003.

Dieckmann, P., Molin Friis, S., Lippert, A., & Østergaard, D. (2009). The art and science of debriefing in simulation: Ideal and practice. *Medical Teacher, 31*(7), e287–94. Retrieved from http://search.ebscohost.com/login.aspx?direct=true&db=rzh&AN=2010396241&site=ehost-live

Dieckmann, P., Gaba, D., & Rall, M. (2007). Deepening the theoretical foundations of patient simulation as social practice. *Simulation in Healthcare: The Journal of the Society for Simulation in Healthcare, 2*, 183–193. doi:10.1097/SIH.0b013e3180f637f5

Diez, N., Rodriguez-Diez, M., Nagore, D., Fernandez, S., Ferrer, M., & Beunza, J. (2013). A randomized trial of cardiopulmonary resuscitation training for medical students: Voice advisory mannequin compared to guidance provided by an instructor. *Simulation in Healthcare: The Journal of the Society for Simulation in Healthcare, 8*, 234–241. doi:10.1097/SIH.0b013e31828e7196

Dobbs, C., Sweitzer, V. & Jeffries, P. (2006). Testing simulation design features using an insulin management simulation in nursing education. *Clinical Simulation in Nursing, 2*(1), e17–e22.

Durham, C. F., Cato, M. L., & Lasater, K. (2014). NLN/Jeffries simulation framework state of the science project: Participant construct. *Clinical Simulation in Nursing, 10*(7), 363–372. doi:10.1016/j.ecns.2014.04.002

Durmaz, A., Dicle, A., Cakan, E., & Cakir, S. (2012). Effect of screen-based computer simulation on knowledge and skill in nursing students' learning of preoperative and postoperative care management: A randomized controlled study. *CIN: Computers, Informatics, Nursing, 30*(4), 196–203. Retrieved from http://search.ebscohost.com/login.aspx?direct=true&db=rzh&AN=2011583355&site=ehost-live

Eaton, M. K., Floyd, K., & Brooks, S. (2011). Student perceptions of simulation's influence on home health and hospice practicum learning. *Clinical Simulation in Nursing,* doi:10.1016/j.ecns.2010.11.003.

Elfrink, V. L., Nininger, J., Rohig, L., & Lee, J. (2009). The case for group planning in human patient simulation. *Nursing Education Perspectives, 30*(2), 83–86.

Fenske, C. L., Harris, M. A., Aebersold, M. L., & Hartman, L. S. (2013). Perception versus reality: A comparative study of the clinical judgment skills of nurses during a simulated activity. *Journal of Continuing Education in Nursing, 44*(9), 399–405. doi:10.3928/00220124-20130701-67

Fero, L. J., O'Donnell, J., Zullo, T. G., Dabbs, A. V., Kitutu, J., Samosky, J. T., & Hoffman, L. A. (2010). Critical thinking skills in nursing students: Comparison of simulation-based performance with metrics. *Journal of Advanced Nursing, 66*(10), 2182–2193. doi:10.1111/j.1365-2648.2010.05385.x

Finan, E., Bismilla, Z., Campbell, C., LeBlanc, V., Jefferies, A., & Whyte, H. E. (2012). Improved procedural performance following a simulation training session may not be transferable to the clinical environment. *Journal of Perinatology, 32*(7), 539–544. doi:10.1038/jp.2011.141

Fisher, D., & King, L. (2013). An integrative literature review on preparing nursing students through simulation to recognize and respond to the deteriorating patient. *Journal of Advanced Nursing, 69*(11), 2375–2388. doi:10.1111/jan.12174

Foster, J. G., Sheriff, S., & Cheney, S. (2008). Using nonfaculty registered nurses to facilitate high-fidelity human patient simulation activities. *Nurse Educator, 33*(3), 137–141.

Retrieved from http://search.ebscohost.com/login.aspx?direct=true&db=rzh&AN=2009932986&site=ehost-live

Fountain, R. A., & Alfred, D. (2009). Student satisfaction with high-fidelity simulation: Does it correlate with learning styles? *Nursing Education Perspectives, 30*(2), 96–98. Retrieved from http://search.ebscohost.com/login.aspx?direct=true&db=rzh&AN=2010258647&site=ehost-live

Fraser, K., Ma, I., Teteris, E., Baxter, H., Wright, B., & McLaughlin, K. (2012). Emotion, cognitive load and learning outcomes during simulation training. *Medical Education, 46*(11), 1055–1062.doi:10.1111/j.1365-2923.2012.04355.x

Garrard, J. (2014). *Health Sciences literature review made easy The matrix method (4th ed.).* Burlington, MA: Jones & Bartlett Learning.

Garrett, B., MacPhee, M., & Jackson, C. (2010). High-fidelity patient simulation: Considerations for effective learning. *Nursing Education Perspectives, 31*(5), 309–313.

Grady, J. L., Kehrer, R. G., Trusty, C. E., Entin, E. B., Entin, E. E., & Brunye, T. T. (2008). Learning nursing procedures: The influence of simulator fidelity and student gender on teaching effectiveness. *Journal of Nursing Education, 47*(9), 403–408. doi:10.3928/01484834-20080901-09

Groom, J. A., Henderson, D., & Sittner, B. J. (2014). NLN/Jeffries simulation framework state of the science project: Simulation design characteristics. *Clinical Simulation in Nursing, 10*(7), 337–344. doi:10.1016/j.ecns.2013.02.004

Guhde, J. (2011). Nursing students' perceptions of the effect on critical thinking, assessment, and learner satisfaction in simple versus complex high-fidelity simulation scenarios. *Journal of Nursing Education, 50*(2), 73–78. doi:10.3928/01484834-20101130-03

Ha, E. (2014). Attitudes toward video-assisted debriefing after simulation in undergraduate nursing students: An application of Q methodology. *Nurse Education Today, 34*(6), 978–984. doi:10.1016/j.nedt.2014.01.003

Hallmark, B., Fentress, Thomas, C. M., & Gantt, L. (2014). The educational practices construct of the NLN/Jeffries simulation framework: State of the science. *Clinical Simulation in Nursing, 10*(7), 345–352. doi:10.1016/j.ecns.2013.04.006

Halstead, J. A., Phillips, J. M., Koller, A., Hardin, K., Porter, M. L., & Dwyer, J. S. (2011). Preparing nurse educators to use simulation technology: A consortium model for practice and education. *Journal of Continuing Education in Nursing, 42*(11), 496–502. doi:10.3928/00220124-20110502-01

Harder, B. N. (2010). Use of simulation in teaching and learning in health sciences: A systematic review. *Journal of Nursing Education, 49*(1), 23–28. doi:10.3928/01484834-20090828-08

Hayden, J. K., Smiley, R. A., Alexander, M., Kardong-Edgren, S., & Jeffries, P. R. (2014). The NCSBN National Simulation Study: A longitudinal, randomized, controlled study replacing clinical hours with simulation in prelicensure nursing education. *Journal of Nursing Regulation, 5*(2S), S1–S63.

Hope, A., Garside, J., & Prescott, S. (2011). Rethinking theory and practice: Pre-registration student nurses experiences of simulation teaching and learning in the acquisition of clinical skills in preparation for practice. *Nurse Education Today, 31*(7), 711–715. doi:10.1016/j.nedt.2010.12.011

Hotchkiss, M. A., Biddle, C., & Fallacaro, M. (2002). Assessing the authenticity of the human simulation experience in anesthesiology. *AANA Journal, 70*(6), 470–473. Retrieved from http://search.ebscohost.com/login.aspx?direct=true&db=rzh&AN=2003035287&site=ehost-live

Howard, V. M., Ross, C., Mitchell, A. M., & Nelson, G. M. (2010). Human patient simulators and interactive case studies: A comparative analysis of learning outcomes and student perceptions. *CIN: Computers, Informatics, Nursing, 28*(1), 42–48. doi:10.1097/NCN.0b013e3181c04939

Ironside, P. M., Jeffries, P. R., & Martin, A. (2009). Fostering patient safety competencies using multiple-patient simulation experiences. *Nursing Outlook, 57*(6), 332–337.

Issenberg, S. B., McGaghie, W. C., Petrusa, E. R., Gordon, D. L., & Scalese, R. J. (2005). Features and uses of high-fidelity medical simulations that lead to effective learning: A BEME systematic review. *Medical Teacher, 27*(1), 10–28. Retrieved from http://search.ebscohost.com/login.aspx?direct=true&db=rzh&AN=2005085405&site=ehost-live

Jeffries, P. R. (2005). A framework for designing, implementing and evaluating simulations used as teaching strategies in nursing. *Nursing Education Perspectives, 26*(2), 96–103.

Jeffries, P. R., & Rogers, K. J. (2012). Theoretical framework for simulation design, In P. R. Jeffries (Ed.), *Simulation in nursing education: From conceptualization to evaluation* (2nd ed., pp. 25–42). New York: National League for Nursing.

Jeffries, P. R., & Rizzolo, M. (2006). Designing and implementing models for the innovative use of simulation to teach nursing care of ill adults and children: A national, multi-site, multi-method study. *National League for Nursing.*

Johannesson, E., Olsson, M., Petersson, G., & Silén, C. (2010). Learning features in computer simulation skills training. *Nurse Education in Practice, 10*(5), 268–273. doi:10.1016/j.nepr.2009.11.018

Jones, A. L., Reese, C. E., & Shelton, D. P. (2014). NLN/Jeffries simulation framework state of the science project: The teacher construct. *Clinical Simulation in Nursing, 10*(7), 353–362. doi:10.1016/j.ecns.2013.10.008

Kaakinen, J., & Arwood, E. (2009). Systematic review of nursing simulation literature for use of learning theory. *International Journal of Nursing Education Scholarship, 6*(1), 1p. doi:10.2202/1548-923X.1688

Kaplan, B. G., Abraham, C., & Gary, R. (2012). Effects of participation vs. observation of a simulation experience on testing outcomes: Implications for logistical planning for a school nursing. *International Journal of Nursing Education Scholarship, 9*(1), 1–15. Retrieved from http://search.ebscohost.com/login.aspx?direct=true&db=rzh&AN=2011630927&site=ehost-live

Kardong-Edgren, S., Starkweather, A. R., & Ward, L. D. (2008). The integration of simulation into a clinical foundations of nursing course: Student and faculty perspectives.

International Journal of Nursing Education Scholarship, 5(1), 1–16.

Karnath, B. M., Das Carlo, M., & Holden, M. D. (2004). A comparison of faculty-led small group learning in combination with computer-based instruction versus computer-based instruction alone on identifying simulated pulmonary sounds. *Teaching & Learning in Medicine, 16*(1), 23–27. Retrieved from http://search.ebscohost.com/login.aspx?direct=true&db=rzh&AN=2005028348&site=ehost-live

Kelly, M. A., Hager, P., & Gallagher, R. (2014). What matters most? students' rankings of simulation components that contribute to clinical judgment. *Journal of Nursing Education, 53*(2), 97–101. doi:10.3928/01484834-20140122-08

Kennedy, C. C., Maldonado, F., & Cook, D. A. (2013). Simulation-based bronchoscopy training: Systematic review and meta-analysis. *Chest, 144*(1), 183–192. doi:10.1378/chest.12-1786

Kiat, T. K., Mei, T. Y., Nagammal, S., & Jonnie, A. (2007). A review of learners' experience with simulation based training in nursing. *Singapore Nursing Journal, 34*(4), 37–43. Retrieved from http://search.ebscohost.com/login.aspx?direct=true&db=rzh&AN=2009753282&site=ehost-live

Kirkpatrick, D. L. (1998). *Evaluating training programs: The four levels.* San Francisco, CA: Bernett-Keehler.

Koskinen, L., Abdelhamid, P., & Likitalo, H. (2008). The simulation method for learning cultural awareness in nursing. *Diversity in Health & Social Care, 5*(1), 55–63. Retrieved from http://search.ebscohost.com/login.aspx?direct=true&db=rzh&AN=2009881225&site=ehost-live

LaFond, C. M., & Vincent, H. V. (2012). A critique of the National League for Nursing/Jeffries Simulation Framework. *Journal of Advanced Nursing, 69*(2), 465–480. doi:10.1111/j.1365-2648.2012.06048.x

Lane, C., & Rollnick, S. (2007). The use of simulated patients and role-play in communication skills training: A review of the literature to August 2005. *Patient Education & Counseling, 67*(1–2), 13–20. Retrieved from http://search.ebscohost.com/login.aspx?direct=true&db=rzh&AN=2009630289&site=ehost-live

Lapkin, S., & Levett-Jones, T. (2011). A cost-utility analysis of medium vs. high-fidelity human patient simulation manikins in nursing education. *Journal of Clinical Nursing, 20*(23), 3543–3552. doi:10.1111/j.1365-2702.2011.03843.x

Leblanc, V. R., Regehr, C., Tavares, W., Scott, A. K., Macdonald, R., & King, K. (2012). The impact of stress on paramedic performance during simulated critical events. *Prehospital & Disaster Medicine, 27*(4), 369–374. Retrieved from http://search.ebscohost.com/login.aspx?direct=true&db=rzh&AN=2011720637&site=ehost-live

LeFlore, J., & Anderson, M. (2009). Alternative educational models for interdisciplinary student teams. *Simulation in Healthcare: The Journal of the Society for Simulation in Healthcare, 4*, 135–142. doi:10.1097/SIH.0b013e318196f839

LeFlore, J., Anderson, M., Zielke, M., Nelson, K., Thomas, P., Hardee, G., & John, L. (2012). Can a virtual patient trainer teach student nurses how to save lives—Teaching nursing students about pediatric respiratory diseases. *Simulation in Healthcare: The Journal of the Society for Simulation in Healthcare, 7*, 10–17. doi:10.1097/SIH.0b013e31823652de

Leigh, G. T. (2008). High-fidelity patient simulation and nursing students' self-efficacy: A review of the literature. *International Journal of Nursing Education Scholarship, 5*(1), 17p. Retrieved from http://search.ebscohost.com/login.aspx?direct=true&db=rzh&AN=2010044624&site=ehost-live

Leighton, K., & Scholl, K. (2009). Simulated codes: understanding the response of undergraduate nursing students. *Clinical Simulation in Nursing, 5*(5), e187–e194.

Levett-Jones, T., & Lapkin, S. (2014). A systematic review of the effectiveness of simulation debriefing in health professional education. *Nurse Education Today, 34*(6), e58–63. doi:10.1016/j.nedt.2013.09.020

Lucisano, K. E., & Talbot, L. A. (2012). Simulation training for advanced airway management for anesthesia and other healthcare providers: A systematic review. *AANA Journal, 80*(1), 25–31. Retrieved from http://search.ebscohost.com/login.aspx?direct=true&db=rzh&AN=2011485353&site=ehost-live

Maran, N. J. and Glavin, R. J. (2003), Low- to high-fidelity simulation – a continuum of medical education?. *Medical Education*, 37: 22–28. doi: 10.1046/j.1365-2923.37.s1.9.x

Marmol, M T., Braga, F. T., Garbin, L. M., Moreli, L., dos Santos, C. B., & de Carvalho, E. C. (2012). Central catheter dressing in a simulator: The effects of tutor's assistance or self-learning tutorial. *Revista Latino-Americana De Enfermagem (RLAE), 20*(6), 1134–1141. doi:S0104-11692012000600016

Matos, F., & Raemer, D. (2013). Mixed-realism simulation of adverse event disclosure: An educational methodology and assessment instrument. *Simulation in Healthcare: The Journal of the Society for Simulation in Healthcare, 8*, 84–90. doi:10.1097/SIH.0b013e31827cbb27

McGaghie, W. C. (2008). Research opportunities in simulation-based medical education using deliberate practice. *Academic Emergency Medicine, 15*(11), 995–1001. Retrieved from http://search.ebscohost.com/login.aspx?direct=true&db=rzh&AN=2010386653&site=ehost-live

McGaghie, W. C., Issenberg, S. B., Petrusa, E. R., & Scalese, R. J. (2006). Effect of practice on standardised learning outcomes in simulation-based medical education. *Medical Education, 40*(8), 792–797. Retrieved from http://search.ebscohost.com/login.aspx?direct=true&db=rzh&AN=2009257333&site=ehost-live

McGaghie, W. C., Issenberg, S. B., Barsuk, J. H., & Wayne, D. B. (2014). A critical review of simulation-based mastery learning with translational outcomes. *Medical Education, 48*(4), 375–385. doi:10.1111/medu.12391

Meakim, C., Boese, T., Decker, S., Franklin, A. E., Gloe, D., Lioce, L., Sando, C. R., & Borum, J. C. (2013). Standards of Best Practice: Simulation Standard I: Terminology. *Clinical Simulation in Nursing, 9*(6S), S3–S11.http://dx.doi.org/10.1016/j.ecns.2013.04.001.

Meyer, M., Connors, H., Hou, Q., & Gajewski, B. (2011). The effect of simulation on clinical performance: A junior nursing student clinical comparison study. *Simulation in Healthcare: The Journal of the Society for Simulation in Healthcare, 6*, 269–277. doi:10.1097/SIH.0b013e318223a048

Montan, K. L., Hreckoviski, B., Dobson, B., Ortenwall, P., Montan, C., Khorram-Manesh, A., Lennquist, L. (2014). Development and evaluation of a new simulation model for interactive training of the medical response to major incidents and disasters. *European Journal of Trauma and Emergency Surgery, 40*(4), 429–443.

Mudumbai, S., Gaba, D., Boulet, J., Howard, S., & Davies, M. (2012). External validation of simulation-based assessments with other performance measures of third-year anesthesiology residents. *Simulation in Healthcare: The Journal of the Society for Simulation in Healthcare, 7*, 73–80. doi:10.1097/SIH.0b013e31823d018a

Nicholson, L. (2012). *The transformational learning process of nursing students during simulated clinical experiences.* D'Youville College. Doctoral dissertation. Retrieved from UMI number 3537521.

Norman, J. (2012). Systematic review of the literature on simulation in nursing education. *ABNF Journal, 23*(2), 24–28. Retrieved from http://search.ebscohost.com/login.aspx?direct=true&db=rzh&AN=2011552819&site=ehost-live

O'Donnell, J. M., Decker, S., Howard, V., Levett-Jones, T., & Miller, C. W. (2014). NLN/Jeffries Simulation Framework state of the science project: Simulation learning outcomes. *Clinical Simulation in Nursing, 10*(7), 373–382. doi:10.1016/j.ecns.2014.06.004

Paige, J. (2014). *Simulation design characteristics: Perspectives held by nurse educators and nursing students.* University of Wisconsin–Milwaukee. Doctoral dissertation. Retrieved from UMI number 3614774.

Paige, J. B., & Morin, K. H. (2013). Simulation fidelity and cueing: A systematic review of the literature. *Clinical Simulation in*

Nursing, 9(11), e481–e489. http://dx.doi. org/10.1016/j.ecns.2013.01.001.

Parker, B. C., & Myrick, F. (2012). The pedagogical ebb and flow of human patient simulation: Empowering through a process of fading support. *Journal of Nursing Education, 51*(7), 365–372. doi:10.3928/ 01484834-20120509-01

Parsh, B. (2010). Characteristics of effective simulated clinical experience instructors: Interviews with undergraduate nursing students. *Journal of Nursing Education, 49*(10), 569–572. doi:10.3928/01484834-20100730-04

Partin, J. L., Payne, T. A., & Slemmons, M. F. (2011). Students' perceptions of their learning experiences using high-fidelity simulation to teach concepts relative to obstetrics. *Nursing Education Perspectives, 32*(3), 186–188. doi:10.5480/1536-5026-32.3.186

Paskins, Z., & Peile, E. (2010). Final year medical students' views on simulation-based teaching: A comparison with the best evidence medical education systematic review. *Medical Teacher, 32*(7), 569–577. doi:10.3109/01421590903544710

Raemer, D., Anderson, M., Cheng, A., Fanning, R., Nadkarni, V., & Savoldelli, G. (2011). Research regarding debriefing as part of the learning process. *Simulation in Healthcare: The Journal of the Society for Simulation in Healthcare, 6*, S52–S57. doi:10.1097/ SIH.0b013e31822724d0

Ravert, P. (2002). An integrative review of computer-based simulation in the education process. *CIN: Computers, Informatics, Nursing, 20*(5), 203–208. Retrieved from http://search.ebscohost.com/login.aspx? direct=true&db=rzh&AN=2002159431&site= ehost-live

Reese, C. E., Jeffries, P. R., & Engum, S. A. (2010). Learning together: using simulations to develop nursing and medical student collaboration. *Nursing Education Perspectives, 31*(1), 33–37.

Rezmer, J., Begaz, T., Treat, R., & Tews, M. (2011). Impact of group size on the effectiveness of a resuscitation simulation curriculum for medical students. *Teaching & Learning in Medicine, 23*(3), 251–255. doi:10.1080/10401334.2011.586920

Roh, Y. S., & Lim, E. J. (2014). Pre-course simulation as a predictor of satisfaction with an emergency nursing clinical course. *International Journal of Nursing Education Scholarship, 11*(1), 1–8. doi:10.1515/ijnes-2013-0083

Rosen, M. A., Hunt, E. A., Pronovost, P. J., Federowicz, M. A., & Weaver, S. J. (2012). In situ simulation in continuing education for the health care professions: A systematic review. *Journal of Continuing Education in the Health Professions, 32*(4), 243–254. doi:10.1002/chp.21152

Rourke, L., Schmidt, M., & Garga, N. (2010). Theory-based research of high fidelity simulation use in nursing education: A review of the literature. *International Journal of Nursing Education Scholarship, 7*(1), 14p. doi:10.2202/1548-923X.1965

Scaringe, J. G., Chen, D., & Ross, D. (2002). The effects of augmented sensory feedback precision on the acquisition and retention of a simulated chiropractic task. *Journal of Manipulative & Physiological Therapeutics, 25*(1), 34–41. Retrieved from http://search.ebscohost.com/login.aspx?direct=true&db= rzh&AN=2002057675&site=ehost-live

Schlairet, M. C., & Fenster, M. J. (2012). Dose and sequence of simulation and direct care experiences among beginning nursing students: A pilot study. *Journal of Nursing Education, 51*(12), 668–675. doi:10.3928/01484834-20121005-03

Schwartz, L. R., Fernandez, R., Kouyoumjian, S. R., Jones, K. A., & Compton, S. (2007). A randomized comparison trial of case-based learning versus human patient simulation in medical student education. *Academic Emergency Medicine, 14*(2), 130–137. Retrieved from http://search.ebscohost.com/login. aspx?direct=true&db=rzh&AN=2009507277 &site=ehost-live

Shanks, D., Brydges, R., den Brok, W., Nair, P., & Hatala, R. (2013). Are two heads better than one? Comparing dyad and self-regulated learning in simulation training. *Medical Education, 47*(12), 1215–1222. doi:10.1111/ medu.12284

Shinnick, M. A., Woo, M., & Evangelista, L. S. (2012). Predictors of knowledge gains using simulation in the education of prelicensure nursing students. *Journal of Professional Nursing, 28*(1), 41–47. doi:10.1016/j.profnurs.2011.06.006

Smith, S. J., & Roehrs, C. J. (2009). High-fidelity simulation: factors correlated with nursing student satisfaction and self-confidence. *Nursing Education Perspectives, 30*(2), 74–78.

Smithburger, P., Kane-Gill, S., Ruby, C., Seybert, M. (2012). Comparing effectiveness of 3 learning strategies: Simulation-based learning, problem-based learning, and standardized patients. *Simulation in Healthcare: The Journal of the Society for Simulation in Healthcare, 7,* 141–146. doi:10.1097/SIH.0b013e31823ee24d

Stegmann, K., Pilz, F., Siebeck, M., & Fischer, F. (2012). Vicarious learning during simulations: Is it more effective than hands-on training? *Medical Education, 46*(10), 1001–1008. doi:10.1111/j.1365-2923.2012.04344.x

Tiffen, J., Corbridge, S., Shen, B. C., & Robinson, P. (2011). Patient simulator for teaching heart and lung assessment skills to advanced practice nursing students. *Clinical Simulation in Nursing, 7*(3), e91–e97.

Tosterud, R., Hedelin, B., & Hall-Lord, M. L. (2013). Nursing students' perceptions of high and low-fidelity simulation used as learning methods. *Nursing Education in Practice, 13,* 262–270.

Trokan-Mathison, N. (2013). *Using simulation to foster the quality and safety education for nurses competencies in associate degree nursing students.* Capella University. Doctoral dissertation. Retrieved from UMI number 3597401.

van Soeren, M., Devlin-Cop, S., MacMillan, K., Baker, L., Egan-Lee, E., & Reeves, S. (2011). Simulated interprofessional education: An analysis of teaching and learning processes. *Journal of Interprofessional Care, 25*(6), 434–440. doi:10.3109/13561820.2011.592229

Walsh, C. M., Sherlock, M. E., Ling, S. C., & Carnahan, H. (2012). Virtual reality simulation training for health professions trainees in gastrointestinal endoscopy. *Cochrane Database of Systematic Reviews,* (6). Retrieved from http://search.ebscohost.com/login.aspx?direct=true&db=rzh&AN=2011632632&site=ehost-live

Waxman, K. T. (2010). The development of evidence-based clinical simulation scenarios: Guidelines for nurse educators. *Journal of Nursing Education, 49*(1), 29–35. doi:10.3928/01484834-20090916-07

Wayne, D., Cohen, E., Singer, B., Moazed, F., Barsuk, J., Lyons, E., Butter, J., & McGaghie, W. (2014). Progress toward improving medical school graduates' skills via a "Boot Camp" curriculum. *Simulation in Healthcare: The Journal of the Society for Simulation in Healthcare, 9,* 33–39. doi:10.1097/SIH.0000000000000001

Weaver, A. (2011). High-fidelity patient simulation in nursing education: An integrative review. *Nursing Education Perspectives, 32*(1), 37–40. doi:10.5480/1536-5026-32.1.37

Wilson, R. D., & Hagler, D. (2012). Through the lens of instructional design: Appraisal of the Jeffries/National League for Nursing Simulation Framework for use in acute care. *Journal of Continuing Education in Nursing, 43*(9), 428–432. doi:10.3928/00220124-20120615-27

Wong, F., Cheung, S., Chung, L., Chan, K., Chan, A., To, T., & Wong, M. (2008). Framework for adopting a problem-based learning approach in a simulated clinical setting. *Journal of Nursing Education, 47*(11), 508–514. doi:10.3928/01484834-20081101-11

Wright, M., Segall, N., Hobbs, G., Phillips-Bute, B., Maynard, L., & Taekman, J. (2013). Standardized assessment for evaluation of team skills: Validity and feasibility. *Simulation in Healthcare: The Journal of the Society for Simulation in Healthcare, 8,* 292–303. doi:10.1097/SIH.0b013e318290a022

Yang, H., Thompson, C., & Bland, M. (2012). Effect of improving the realism of simulated clinical judgment tasks on nurses' overconfidence and under confidence: Evidence from a comparative confidence calibration analysis. *International Journal of Nursing Studies, 49*(12), 1505–1511. doi:10.1016/j.ijnurstu.2012.08.005

Young, K. P., & Shellenbarger, T. (2012). Interpreting the NLN Jeffries Framework in the context of nurse educator preparation. *Journal of Nursing Education, 51*(8), 422–428.

Yuan, H. B., Williams, B. A., & Fang, J. B. (2012). The contribution of high-fidelity simulation to nursing students' confidence and competence: A systematic review. *International Nursing Review, 59*(1), 26–33. doi:10.1111/j.1466-7657.2011.00964.x

Yuan, H. B., Williams, B. A., Fang, J. B., & Ye, Q. H. (2012). A systematic review of selected evidence on improving knowledge and skills through high-fidelity simulation. *Nurse Education Today, 32*(3), 294–298. doi:10.1016/j.nedt.2011.07.010

Zulkosky, K. D. (2012). Simulation use in the classroom: impact on knowledge acquisition, satisfaction and self-confidence. *Clinical Simulation in Nursing, 8*(1), e25–e33.

Annotations on Key References

▸ Brewer (2011, p. 315) identified studies and recommended educational techniques for simulation.

▸ Cook et al. (2013) completed a systematic review that largely confirmed the features of effective simulation first described by Issenberg et al. (2005) and added additional features.

▸ Issenberg et al. (2005) completed a BEME Review describing features and uses of high-fidelity simulations that lead to effective learning.

▸ Kaakinen and Arwood (2009) provide a systematic review of the literature related to the use of learning theory in nursing simulation research.

▸ McGaghie et al. (2014) use the critical review technique to describe the state of simulation-based mastery learning and its contributions to educational outcomes, improved patient care, patient outcomes, cost savings, and "systemic educational and patient care improvements" (p. 377).

▸ Waxman (2010) describes guidelines for creating evidence-based simulation scenarios.

▸ Weinger (2010) uses concepts from pharmacology to describe a framework that can guide research aimed at establishing the evidence base for simulation design and implementation.

3

NLN Jeffries Simulation Theory: Brief Narrative Description

Pamela R. Jeffries, PhD, RN, FAAN, ANEF
Beth Rodgers, PhD, RN, FAAN
Katie Anne Adamson, PhD, RN

Based on the thorough synthesis of the literature and discussion among simulation researchers and leaders, the NLN Jeffries Simulation framework (2005, 2007, 2012) is now referred to as the NLN Jeffries Simulation Theory with a few minor changes within the conceptual illustration. In this chapter, the concepts of this theory are briefly described to provide more clarity and to explain Figure 3.1 and the new NLN Jeffries Simulation Theory.

CONTEXT

Contextual factors such as *circumstances* and *setting* impact every aspect of the simulation and are an important starting point in designing or evaluating simulation. The *context* may include the place (academic vs. practice; in-situ vs. lab) and the overarching purpose of the simulation, for example, whether the simulation is for evaluation or instructional purposes.

BACKGROUND

Within this *context,* the **background** includes the goal(s) of the simulation and specific expectations or benchmarks that influence the **design** of the simulation. The theoretical perspective for the specific **simulation experience** and how the simulation fits within the larger curriculum are all important elements of the background and inform the simulation design and implementation. Finally, the background of a simulation includes resources such as time and equipment, as well as how these resources will be allocated.

DESIGN

Outside of and preceding the actual simulation experience are specific elements that make up the simulation design. Although some elements of the simulation design may

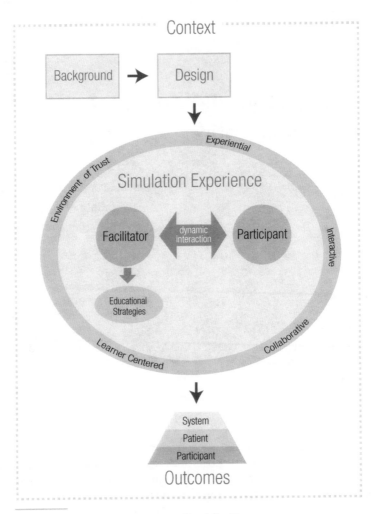

FIGURE 3.1 Diagram of NLN Jeffries Simulation Theory.

be changed during implementation of the simulation experience, there are aspects of the design that need to be considered in preparation for the simulation experience. The design includes the specific learning objectives that guide the development or selection of activities and scenario(s) with appropriate content and problem-solving complexity. Elements of physical and conceptual fidelity—including decisions about equipment, moulage (physical), and appropriate, predetermined *facilitator* responses to *participants'* interventions (conceptual)—are established as part of the simulation design. Participant and observer roles (including whether or not videography will be used), progression of activities, and briefing/debriefing strategies are all established as part of the simulation design.

SIMULATION EXPERIENCE

The simulation experience is characterized by an environment that is experiential, inter-active, collaborative, and learner centered. This environment requires the establish-ment of trust; both the facilitator and participant share responsibility for maintaining this environment. They enhance the quality of the simulation experience through "buying-in" to the authenticity of the experience and suspending disbelief. This helps promote engagement and psychological fidelity within the simulation experience (Kiat, Mei, Nagammal, & Jonnie, 2007; Leighton & Sholl, 2009; van Soeren et al., 2011).

FACILITATOR AND EDUCATIONAL STRATEGIES

Within this simulation experience is a dynamic interaction between the facilitator and the participant. The literature about the characteristics these individuals bring to the simula-tion experience and how they affect the simulation experience is extensive. Facilitator attributes include (but are not limited to) skill, educational techniques, and preparation (Parsh, 2010; Parker & Myrick, 2012). The facilitator responds to emerging participant needs during the simulation experience by adjusting educational strategies such as altering the planned progression and timing of activities and providing appropriate feedback in the form of cues (during) and debriefing (toward the end) of the simulation experience.

PARTICIPANT

Participant attributes also affect the simulation learning experience. The literature describes attributes that are innate to the participant such as age (Fenske, Harris, Aebersold, & Hartman, 2013), gender (Diez et al., 2013), level of anxiety (Leblanc et al., 2012; Beischel, 2013), and self-confidence (Jeffries & Rogers, 2012) as well as modifiable attributes such as pre-paredness for the simulation (Beischel, 2011). Many elements of the simulation design such as role assignment affect individual participants and may impact their learning experience (Kaplan, Abraham, & Gary, 2012).

OUTCOMES

Finally, outcomes of the simulation may be separated into three areas: participant, patient (or care recipient), and system outcomes. The literature largely focuses on par-ticipant outcomes including reaction (satisfaction, self-confidence), learning (changes in knowledge, skills, attitudes), and behavior (how learning transfers to the clinical envi-ronment). However, there is emerging literature about outcomes of simulation covering health outcomes of patients or care recipients whose caregivers were trained using simulation and organizational/system outcomes of simulation, including studies about cost-effectiveness and changes of practice. Figure 3.1 depicts outcomes in a triangu-lar format based on the hierarchy of outcomes with participant, patient, and system outcomes as defined and extracted from the body of literature found on simulation outcomes.

References

Beischel, K. P. (2011). Variables affecting learning in a simulation experience: A mixed methods study. *Western Journal of Nursing Research, 35*(2), 226–247.

Diez, N., Rodriguez-Diez, M., Nagore, D., Fernandez, S., Ferrer, M., & Beunza, J. (2013). A randomized trial of cardiopulmonary resuscitation training for medical students: Voice advisory mannequin compared to guidance provided by an instructor. *Simulation in Healthcare: The Journal of the Society for Simulation in Healthcare, 8,* 234–241. doi:10.1097/SIH.0b013e31828e7196

Fenske, C. L., Harris, M. A., Aebersold, M. L., & Hartman, L. S. (2013). Perception versus reality: A comparative study of the clinical judgment skills of nurses during a simulated activity. *Journal of Continuing Education in Nursing, 44*(9), 399–405. doi:10.3928/00220124-20130701-67

Jeffries, P. R. (2005). A framework for designing, implementing, and evaluating simulations used as teaching strategies in nursing. *Nursing Education Perspectives, 26*(2): 96–103.

Jeffries, P. R. (Ed.). (2007). *Simulation in nursing education: From conceptualization to evaluation.* New York: National League for Nursing.

Jeffries, P. R. (Ed.). (2012). *Simulation in nursing education: From conceptualization to evaluation* (2nd ed.). New York: National League for Nursing.

Jeffries, P. R., & Rogers, K. J. (2012). Theoretical framework for simulation design/ In P. R. Jeffries (Ed.), *Simulation in nursing education: From conceptualization to evaluation* (2nd ed., pp. 25-42). New York: National League for Nursing.

Kaplan, B. G., Abraham, C., & Gary, R. (2012). Effects of participation vs. observation of a simulation experience on testing outcomes: Implications for logistical planning for a school nursing. *International Journal of Nursing Education Scholarship, 9*(1), 1–15. Retrieved from http://search.ebscohost.com/login.aspx?direct=true&db=rzh&AN=2011630927&site=ehost-live

Kiat, T. K., Mei, T. Y., Nagammal, S., & Jonnie, A. (2007). A review of learners' experience with simulation based training in nursing. *Singapore Nursing Journal, 34*(4), 37–43. Retrieved from http://search.ebscohost.com/login.aspx?direct=true&db=rzh&AN=2009753282&site=ehost-live

Leblanc, V. R., Regehr, C., Tavares, W., Scott, A. K., Macdonald, R., & King, K. (2012). The impact of stress on paramedic performance during simulated critical events. *Prehospital & Disaster Medicine, 27*(4), 369–374. Retrieved from http://search.ebscohost.com/login.aspx?direct=true&db=rzh&AN=2011720637&site=ehost-live

Leighton, K., & Scholl, K. (2009). Simulated codes: understanding the response of undergraduate nursing students. *Clinical Simulation in Nursing, 5*(5), e187–e194.

Parsh, B. (2010). Characteristics of effective simulated clinical experience instructors: Interviews with undergraduate nursing students. *Journal of Nursing Education, 49*(10), 569–572. doi:10.3928/01484834-20100730-04

Parker, B. C., & Myrick, F. (2012). The pedagogical ebb and flow of human patient simulation: Empowering through a process of fading support. *Journal of Nursing Education, 51*(7), 365–372. doi:10.3928/01484834-20120509-01

van Soeren, M., Devlin-Cop, S., MacMillan, K., Baker, L., Egan-Lee, E., & Reeves, S. (2011). Simulated interprofessional education: An analysis of teaching and learning processes. *Journal of Interprofessional Care, 25*(6), 434–440. doi:10.3109/13561820.2011.592229

4

NLN Vision: Teaching with Simulation

Susan Gross Forneris, PhD, RN, CNE, CHSE-A

Mary Fey, PhD, RN, CHSE

The realities of the changing health care system, health care reform, and technological advances in health care delivery are driving change in nursing curricula. The health care environment has become more complex and more diverse, with an emphasis on shorter inpatient hospital stays and a shift from inpatient to outpatient and community health care (Institute of Medicine [IOM], 2011). The increasing complexity of the health care environment demands the use of new theory-based approaches to the education of nurses. Content-laden curricula that transmit contextualized information alone do not sufficiently prepare students for the realities of practice. Simulation is an evidence-based teaching methodology that is grounded in theory from diverse fields, including education, cognitive psychology, and adult learning. Consistent with the need for "radical transformation" in nursing education, as described in the Carnegie Report for the Advancement of Teaching (Benner, Stuphen, Leonard & Day, 2010), simulation provides a means for teaching that is situated in the context of practice. Simulation is a contextual teaching methodology, providing for the application of theoretical knowledge as nursing students develop their clinical reasoning skills in environments that closely replicate actual practice and pose no risk to patients—an important factor driving the rapid adoption of simulation in nursing education.

Schools of nursing are examining their curricula to determine how they might make changes to better achieve the goal of creating nurses skilled in multiple ways of thinking, including clinical reasoning and critical reflection (Benner et al., 2010). The use of evidence guiding both practice and education shifts the focus to teaching *with and about context* to better prepare students for the realities that they will face in practice. The NLN Jeffries theory provides guidance to both educators and researchers as they continue to develop simulation's potential as a powerful teaching methodology.

For more than a decade, the NLN has promoted simulation as a teaching methodology to prepare nurses for practice across the continuum of care in today's complex health care environment. That experience—reinforced by the League's mission to promote excellence in nursing education for building a strong and diverse nursing workforce to advance the health of our nation and the global community, along with core values of caring, integrity, diversity, and excellence—furnishes a strong foundation to address the challenges and opportunities arising from the use of simulation in nursing education. To that end, the National League for Nursing Board of Governors published a vision statement for teaching simulation in April 2015 (NLN, 2015). This statement, *A Vision for Teaching with Simulation,* is presented below.

INTRODUCTION

Simulation can take many forms, including human patient simulation using manikins and/or standardized patients, virtual and computer-based simulations, simulation done to teach psychomotor skills, or role play (Society for Simulation in Healthcare, 2015). Simulation provides a rich learning opportunity for students to integrate theory with practice while making real-time clinical decisions in an environment that poses no risk to patients.

The National Council of State Boards of Nursing (NCSBN) landmark, multi-site, longitudinal study explored the role and outcomes of simulation in prelicensure clinical nursing education in the United States (Hayden, Smiley, Alexander, Kardong-Edgren, & Jeffries, 2014). The NLN endorses the study findings, which concluded that there is substantial evidence that simulation can be substituted for up to 50 percent of traditional clinical experiences under conditions comparable to those described in the study (NLN, 2014).

Simulation creates transformational learning experience for all nursing students and provides diverse perspectives on caring for patients across the continuum of care. Learning in simulation allows for situated cognition—or learning in context—a concept at the forefront of contemporary educational reform. As teachers and learners move away from content-laden curricula to curricula that emphasize experiential learning, it is critical that nurse educators have the requisite knowledge and skills to use simulation to its full potential. Experience followed by learner self-reflection is core to all methods.

BACKGROUND AND SIGNIFICANCE

In 2003, the NLN conducted the landmark simulation study "Designing and Implementing Models for the Innovative Use of Simulation to Teach Nursing Care of Ill Adults and Children: A National Multi-Site, Multi-Method Study" (Jeffries & Rizzolo, 2007). This study resulted in the development of the NLN Jeffries Simulation Framework, widely used as the theoretical foundation for research in simulation use and efficacy, both nationally and internationally. Since then, the NLN published a revised version of the framework (Jeffries and Rogers, 2012) and developed and disseminated many tools to help faculty teach with simulation:

▸ The Simulation Innovation and Resource Center (SIRC; sirc.nln.org) a comprehensive website providing education and support to advance simulation in nursing education, was launched in 2007.

▸ More than 50 evidence-based simulation scenarios that guide faculty use of simulation throughout schools of nursing in the United States and around the world.

▸ The Leadership Development Program for Simulation Educators began in 2011; more than 100 simulation leaders have participated in the program.

Recent advances in simulation technology and pedagogy allow nurse educators to facilitate experiential learning in ways unimaginable when the first patient simulator, "Mrs. Chase," was delivered to the Hartford Hospital Training School for Nurses in 1911. Today, simulation is more than a way to teach and practice psychomotor skills. It is an evidence-based strategy to facilitate high-quality experiences that foster thinking and clinical reasoning skills for students. The emphasis is on creating contextual learning environments that replicate crucial practice situations. Now more than ever— with changes in health care access and technological advances in health care delivery, the increasing complexity of patient care, and the growing lack of clinical placements for students—it is imperative to embed quality simulation experiences throughout the program of learning.

Practice Trends Influencing the Use of Simulation in Nursing Education

▸ Data confirming medical errors have driven *patient safety* to the forefront of health care reform. Through the incorporation of concepts from the Quality and Safety Education for Nurses (QSEN) initiative (Cronenwett, Sherwood, & Gelmon, 2009), nursing education is placing more emphasis on teaching the importance of patient safety. The literature supports that simulation-based education with deliberate practice is effective in achieving specific clinical goals related to patient safety (McGaghie, Issenberg, Cohen, Barsuk, & Wayne, 2011).

▸ *Interprofessional education* and collaborative practice are seen as key in achieving safe, high-quality, accessible, patient-centered care. Simulation that is focused on interprofessional learning objectives provides the opportunity for nursing students to learn with, from, and about their peers in other health care disciplines (Interprofessional Education Collaborative, 2011).

Factors Informing the Expanded and Consistent Use of Simulation

▸ Passive learning approaches are being replaced by *experiential learning,* that is, active learning approaches whereby students become the center of the teaching and change from mere consumers of education to engaged active learners (Jeffries & Clochesy, 2012). Unique challenges exist for the educator to devise teaching strategies that move from highly structured to self-directed learning and reactive thinking to critically reflective proactive thinking. Contextualized learning brings classroom and clinical together; simulation engages learners with diverse perspectives to reflect and reframe the understanding of practice, bringing thinking and doing together.

▸ Schools of nursing are increasingly challenged to provide high-quality *clinical experiences* for students. Educators have turned to simulation as a way to provide rich learning experiences that can replicate actual clinical experiences. Simulation can standardize clinical experiences in this time of unpredictable and often unequal clinical learning opportunities. The NCSBN study (Hayden et al., 2014) highlights simulation's success as a teaching tool, for example, student achievement on content-focused, end-of-course exams, and their development of clinical reasoning skills similar to those achieved in traditional clinical experiences.

▸ *Guidelines and quality measures* for simulation programs and facilitators have been published by both the International Nursing Association for Clinical Simulation and Learning (INACSL) and the Society for Simulation in Healthcare (SSH). The INACSL standards (2013) provide guidance on terminology, the professional integrity of participants, participant objectives, the facilitator, facilitation, debriefing, and participant assessment and evaluation. SSH standards relate to the certification of health care simulation educators (SSH, 2012) and the accreditation of simulation centers (SSH, 2014).

> It is important to *evaluate simulation programs and facilitators* for their ability to support program outcomes and organizational goals. Used to drive continuous quality improvement, three evaluation perspectives are valuable when assessing the quality of simulation-based education:

   ■ Evaluation of individual simulation experiences by both faculty and learners ensures that the simulation experience contributes to meeting course and/or program outcomes.

   ■ Evaluation of the simulation program helps underpin the integration of simulation into a nursing curriculum as a whole.

   ■ Evaluation of the simulation facilitator affects the quality of the simulation experience and validates the competence of the facilitator.

> Evaluation of learning outcomes along with evaluation of the simulation facilitator is accomplished using *reliable and valid instruments.* Though existing published instruments with psychometrics should be used when appropriate (Adamson, Kardong-Edgren, & Willhaus, 2013), simulation programs may choose to create their own if no previously validated tools exist to accomplish their objective. Ensuring the validity and reliability of the instrument is integral to the development process; instruments that lack them should not be used.

> Standards of practice, accreditation standards, and evidence from NCSBN make it clear that simulation requires *specialized faculty development resources.* The creation of simulation programs should include the development of simulation leaders to help faculty integrate the programs into the curriculum. Also critical are resources for faculty development, allocation of faculty workload hours to support best practices, and the provision of an appropriately realistic environment (Jeffries, Dreifuerst, Kardong-Edgren, Hayden, 2015).

> Curricular changes should include curriculum maps and blueprints to be used by **simulation teams** of faculty (Jeffries, Driefuerst, Kardong-Edgren, & Hayden, 2015). Responsible for developing, facilitating, and evaluating the experience, these teams use specific skills to create a realistic and pedagogically sound experience using an applicable theory or framework. When guiding the simulation experience and subsequent debriefing, faculty should provide formative or summative evaluation of simulation participants. In order for nurse educators to meet these responsibilities, additional personnel are needed to provide administrative and operational support.

> Simulation and debriefing teaching techniques are not limited to clinical encounters in the simulation laboratory. As faculty teams bring case studies to life in the classroom with virtual simulations, standardized patients, and human patient simulators, they can facilitate simulation and debriefing that supports didactic content. Similarly, the *use of theory-based debriefing* enhances the educator's ability to assess learning needs and close performance gaps in multiple settings (Hayden et al., 2014).

CALL TO ACTION

The increasing body of evidence supporting the effectiveness of simulation in health care education engenders a call to action. The NLN has identified key strategies and resources to address the need for a more contextual, experiential type of learning through simulation. Links to these resources are found in the full text of the NLN Vision statement online: http://www.nln.org/about/position-statements/nln-living-documents:

> ▶ Core and advanced courses in simulation for faculty to acquire the foundational knowledge needed to begin using simulations as a valuable learning tool are available on the SIRC.
> ▶ The NLN Advancing Care Excellence for Seniors (ACE.S) and for Veterans (ACE.V— web pages offer free teaching-ready unfolding cases based in simulation.
> ▶ Collaborative efforts have resulted in the creation of simulation scenario sets and a virtual simulation product: vSim for Nursing.
> ▶ Two debriefing courses for faculty are offered through the SIRC, as well as an annotated bibliography focused on recent advances in simulation debriefing techniques and outcomes.
> ▶ The NLN's Leadership Institute offers a yearlong leadership program for simulation educators.

RECOMMENDATIONS

For Deans, Directors, Chairs of Nursing Programs

> ▶ Create strategic partnerships with schools and clinical agencies to capitalize on shared simulation resources.
> ▶ Ensure an adequate number of dedicated simulation faculty with training and expertise in the pedagogy of simulation.
> ▶ Include operational support staff as a part of the simulation team.
> ▶ Budget annually for faculty development in simulation pedagogy and theory-based debriefing.
> ▶ Support the development of simulation leaders among the faculty.

For Nurse Faculty

> ▶ Purposefully integrate simulation into the curriculum with clear connections toward achievement of student learning outcomes.
> ▶ Incorporate simulation standards of practice in the design, implementation, and evaluation of simulation-based experiences.
> ▶ Use evidence-based resources consistently to ensure competence in debriefing.
> ▶ Partner with faculty from other disciplines to create interprofessional simulation experiences.
> ▶ Pursue the development of expertise as a simulation leader.

For the NLN

> Provide professional development resources for faculty to:
> - Incorporate standards of practice in simulation pedagogy and theory-based debriefing
> - Integrate simulation into nursing curricula
> - Enhance faculty expertise in the use of theory-based debriefing in simulation
> - Evaluate simulation experiences using valid and reliable instruments

> Collaborate with key stakeholders (e.g., INACSL, SSH, NCSBN, Laerdal, Wolters Kluwer) to develop and disseminate best practices in the use of simulation in teaching and learning and integrating debriefing into learning activities throughout the curriculum to better engage students in the learning process.

> Provide opportunities for the development of simulation research scholars through the NLN Center for Innovation in Simulation and Technology.

> Increase support of multi-site research studies in simulation pedagogy.

> Partner with simulation scholars and nurse theorists to study and further develop the NLN Jeffries Simulation Theory.

References

Adamson, K. A., Kardong-Edgren, S., & Willhaus, J. (2013). An updated review of published simulation evaluation instruments. *Clinical Simulation in Nursing, 9*(9), e393–e400.

Benner, P., Sutphen, M., Leonard, V., & Day, L. (2010). *Educating nurses: A call for radical transformation*. San Francisco, CA: Jossey-Bass.

Cronenwett, L., Sherwood, G., & Gelmon, S. B. (2009). Improving quality and safety education: The QSEN Learning Collaborative. *Nursing Outlook, 57*(6), 304–312.

Hayden, J. K., Smiley, R. A., Alexander, M., Kardong-Edgren, S., & Jeffries, P. R. (2014). Supplement: The NCSBN National Simulation Study: A longitudinal, randomized, controlled study replacing clinical hours with simulation in prelicensure nursing education. *Journal of Nursing Regulation, 5*(2), S1–S64.

International Nursing Association for Clinical Simulation and Learning. (2013). *Standards of best practice: Simulation*. Retrieved from http://www.inacsl.org/files/journal/Complete% 202013%20Standards.pdf

Institute of Medicine (IOM). (2011). *The future of nursing: Leading change, advancing health*. Washington, DC: National Academies Press.

Interprofessional Education Collaborative. (2011). Core competencies for interprofessional collaborative practice. Retrieved from https://ipecollaborative.org/Resources.html

Jeffries, P. R., & Clochesy, J. M. (2012). Clinical simulations: An experiential, student-centered pedagogical approach. In D. M. Billings & J. A. Halstead (Eds). *Teaching in nursing: A guide for faculty* (4th ed., pp. 352–368). St. Louis, MO: Elsevier Health Sciences.

Jeffries, P. R., Dreifuerst, K. T., Kardong-Edgren, S., & Hayden, J. (2015). Faculty development when initiating simulation programs: Lessons learned from the National Simulation Study. *Journal of Nursing Regulation, 5*(4), 17–23.

Jeffries, P. R., & Rizzolo, M. A. (2007). Designing and implementing models for the innovative use of simulation to teach nursing care of ill adults and children: A national, multi-site, multi-method study [Summary

Report]. In P. R. Jeffries (Ed.), *Simulation in nursing education: From conceptualization to evaluation* (Appendix A, pp. 147–159). New York, NY: National League for Nursing.

Jeffries, P. R., & Rogers, K. J. (2012). Theoretical framework for simulation design. In P. R. Jeffries (Ed.), *Simulation in nursing education: From conceptualization to evaluation* (2nd ed., pp. 25–41). New York, NY: National League for Nursing.

McGaghie, W. C., Issenberg, S. B., Cohen, M. E. R., Barsuk, J. H., & Wayne, D. B. (2011). Does simulation-based medical education with deliberate practice yield better results than traditional clinical education? A meta-analytic comparative review of the evidence. *Academic Medicine, 86*(6), 706.

National League for Nursing (NLN). (2014). NLN response to NCSBN simulation study. Retrieved from http://www.nln.org/docs/default-source/about/nln-vision-series-%28position-statements%29/ncsbnstudy responsefinal.pdf?sfvrsn=4

National League for Nursing (NLN). (2015). A vision for teaching with simulation. [NLN Vision Series]. Retrieved from http://www.nln.org/docs/default-source/about/nln-vision-series-%28position-statements%29/vision-statement-a-vision-for-teaching-with-simulation.pdf?sfvrsn=0

Society for Simulation in Healthcare (SSH). (2012). *Certification standards and elements.* Retrieved from http://www.ssih.org/Portals/48/Certification/CHSE%20 Standards.pdf

Society for Simulation in Healthcare (SSH). (2014). *Accreditation standards.* Retrieved from http://www.ssih.org/Portals/48/Accreditation/14_A_Standards.pdf

Society for Simulation in Healthcare (SSH). (2015). *About simulation.* Retrieved from http://www.ssih.org/About-Simulation

5

Future Research and Next Steps

Pamela R. Jeffries, PhD, RN, FAAN, ANEF
Katie Anne Adamson, PhD, RN
Beth Rodgers, PhD, RN, FAAN

PRIORITY AREAS FOR RESEARCH

While the focus of this systematic review related to the use of the NLN Jeffries Simulation Framework was to discuss the recurring themes, gaps, and key issues, as well as summarize what currently constitutes the best practices and what current research supports, it was hard not to simultaneously identify priority areas in which research is needed. In fact, within the document of bulleted items pulled directly from the literature addressing the objectives of the review, ideas for priority areas in which research is needed took up no less than 25% of the space. Clearly, researchers are not satisfied with the current state of the science around simulation. The following outlines the top research priorities extracted from the current literature and state of the science.

> - What are the unintended consequences of simulation training? (Owen, 2014)

> - Is simulation cost-effective and how can educational practices and simulation design characteristics be manipulated to optimize the cost-effectiveness equation? (Kennedy, Maldonado, & Cook, 2013; Weaver, 2011).

> - Do gains from simulation last and do they translate into improved outcomes? There is a need for longitudinal data about the efficacy of simulation and skill decay (McGaghie, 2008; Yeung, Dubrowski, & Carnahan, 2013; Finan et al., 2012; Weaver, 2011).

> - What are the impacts of deliberate practice and mastery learning? There is a need for randomized controlled trials using deliberate practice and mastery learning (McGaghie, 2008).

> - Improved measurement practices and research designs, including better interpretations of statistical and clinical significance of findings (Harder, 2010; LeFlore et al., 2012; McGaghie, 2008; Yuan, Williams & Fang, 2012; Yeung et al., 2013)

> - The relationships between confidence/self-efficacy, knowledge gains, competence/performance, and patient outcomes (Burke, 2010; Dobbs, Sweitzer, & Jeffries, 2006; Hauber, Cormier, & Whyte, 2010; McGaghie, 2008; Rosen et al., 2012; Tiffen, Corbridge, Shen, & Robinson, 2011; Wilson & Hagler, 2012)

> Determining what are "good" educational practices and whether simulation or other educational practices make simulation effective (Hallenbeck, 2012). Determining which scenarios are more effective: simple or complex (Guhde, 2011; Parker & Myrick, 2012). Determining which lab is more effective: virtual or skill (Durmaz, Dicle, Cakan, & Cakir, 2012; Ravert, 2002).

> Determining what characteristics of debriefing are most effective for specified desired outcomes (Bond et al., 2006; Levett-Jones & Lapkin, 2014)

> Determining whether simulation be effectively delivered at a distance (Berg, Wong, & Vincent, 2007)

> How long should a simulation run? What are the determining factors that ultimately affect the amount of time a simulation should be implemented with participants? Is there a set amount of time that should be strived for when creating and implementing a high-quality simulation?

> There is a need for testing additional conceptual frameworks, including "10 rights of simulation" suggested by Weinger (2010).

> Can the notion of fidelity be clarified and standardized so that evidence regarding best practices related to fidelity can be identified?

> Organizationally, what recommendations or best practices can be supported by empirical data? Simulation facilitator training, facilities, equipment, and technology support are all important components of a simulation program, but few best practices have been established (Bremner, Aduddell, Bennett, & VanGeest, 2006; Cant & Cooper, 2010; Childs & Sepples, 2006; Howard, Englert, Kameg, & Perozzi, 2011).

SUMMARY

This monograph serves as a tool and guide for conducting research for all nurse educators and researchers interested in clinical simulations, best practices, and discovering new knowledge and practices in this clinical arena of education. The theory serves to articulate phenomena and their relationships to guide practice in the arena of simulations. The challenge is now to test and use this theory to guide research in studying the simulation phenomena and contribute to the science of nursing education. As stated previously, much of the simulation research is still in embryonic stages, but providing a mid-range theory to study the phenomena can only facilitate the discovery of best practices, outcomes, and systems change through the research and development of new knowledge and practices. Additional research and evaluation are crucial in advancing theory and science in any area of interest. New findings based on the conduct of research using this theory, and the evaluation of its implementation in applied settings, will contribute to further development of the theory and advancement of the science of simulation in a focused and systematic manner (Rodgers, 2005).

References

Berg, B. W., Wong, L., & Vincent, D. S. (2007). Teaching nursing skills at a distance using a remotely controlled human patient simulator. *Journal of Telemedicine & Telecare,*

13, S3:17–9. Retrieved from http://search.ebscohost.com/login.aspx?direct=true&db=rzh&AN=2009874249&site=ehost-live

Bond, W. F., Deitrick, L. M., Eberhardt, M., Barr, G. C., Kane, B. G., Worrilow, C. C.,... Croskerry, P. (2006). Cognitive versus technical debriefing after simulation training. *Academic Emergency Medicine, 13*(3), 276–283. Retrieved from http://search.ebscohost.com/login.aspx?direct=true&db=rzh&AN=2009231674&site=ehost-live

Bremner, M. N., Aduddell, K., Bennett, D. N., & VanGeest, J. B. (2006). The use of human patient simulators: Best practices with novice nursing students. *Nurse Educator, 31*(4), 170–174. Retrieved from http://search.ebscohost.com/login.aspx?direct=true&db=rzh&AN=2009251311&site=ehost-live

Burke, P. M. (2010). A simulation case study from an instructional design framework. *Teaching & Learning in Nursing, 5*(2), 73–77. doi:10.1016/j.teln.2010.01.003

Cant, R. P., & Cooper, S. J. (2010). Simulation-based learning in nurse education: Systematic review. *Journal of Advanced Nursing, 66*(1), 3–15. doi:10.1111/j.1365-2648.2009.05240.x

Childs, J. C., & Sepples, S. (2006). Clinical teaching by simulation: lessons learned from a complex patient care scenario. *Nursing Education Perspectives, 27*(3), 154–158.

Dobbs, C., Sweitzer, V., & Jeffries, P. (2006). Testing simulation design features using an insulin management simulation in nursing education. *Clinical Simulation in Nursing, 2*(1), e17–e22.

Durmaz, A., Dicle, A., Cakan, E., & Cakir, S. (2012). Effect of screen-based computer simulation on knowledge and skill in nursing students' learning of preoperative and postoperative care management: A randomized controlled study. *CIN: Computers, Informatics, Nursing, 30*(4), 196–203. Retrieved from http://search.ebscohost.com/login.aspx?direct=true&db=rzh&AN=2011583355&site=ehost-live

Finan, E., Bismilla, Z., Campbell, C., LeBlanc, V., Jefferies, A., & Whyte, H., E. (2012). Improved procedural performance following a simulation training session may not be transferable to the clinical environment. *Journal of Perinatology, 32*(7), 539–544. doi:10.1038/jp.2011.141

Hallenbeck, V. J. (2012). Use of high-fidelity simulation for staff education/development: A systematic review of the literature. *Journal for Nurses in Staff Development, 28*(6), 260. doi:10.1097/NND.0b013e31827259c7

Harder, B. N. (2010). Use of simulation in teaching and learning in health sciences: A systematic review. *Journal of Nursing Education, 49*(1), 23–28. doi:10.3928/01484834-20090828-08

Hauber, R. P., Cormier, E., & Whyte I. J. (2010). An exploration of the relationship between knowledge and performance-related variables in high-fidelity simulation: Designing instruction that promotes expertise in practice. *Nursing Education Perspectives, 31*(4), 242–246. Retrieved from http://search.ebscohost.com/login.aspx?direct=true&db=rzh&AN=2010913909&site=ehost-live

Howard, V. M., Englert, N., Kameg, K., & Perozzi, K. (2011). Integration of simulation across the undergraduate curriculum: Student and faculty perspectives. *Clinical Simulation in Nursing, 7*(1), e1–e10. doi:10.1016/j.ecns.2009.10.004

Kennedy, C. C., Maldonado, F., & Cook, D. A. (2013). Simulation-based bronchoscopy training: Systematic review and meta-analysis. *Chest, 144*(1), 183–192. doi:10.1378/chest.12-1786

LeFlore, J., Anderson, M., Zielke, M., Nelson, K., Thomas, P., Hardee, G., & John, L. (2012). Can a virtual patient trainer teach student nurses how to save lives—Teaching nursing students about pediatric respiratory diseases. *Simulation in Healthcare: The Journal of the Society for Simulation in Healthcare, 7*, 10–17. doi:10.1097/SIH.0b013e31823652de

Levett-Jones, T., & Lapkin, S. (2014). A systematic review of the effectiveness of simulation debriefing in health professional education. *Nurse Education Today, 34*(6), e58–63. doi:10.1016/j.nedt.2013.09.020

McGaghie, W. C. (2008). Research opportunities in simulation-based medical education using deliberate practice. *Academic*

Emergency Medicine, 15(11), 995–1001. Retrieved from http://search.ebscohost. com/login.aspx?direct=true&db=rzh&AN= 2010386653&site=ehost-live

Owen, H. (2014). Unexpected consequences of simulator use in medical education: A cautionary tale. *Simulation in Healthcare: The Journal of the Society for Simulation in Healthcare, 9*, 149–152. doi:10.1097/ SIH.0000000000000014

Parker, B. C., & Myrick, F. (2012). The pedagogical ebb and flow of human patient simulation: Empowering through a process of fading support. *Journal of Nursing Education, 51*(7), 365–372. doi:10.3928/01484834-20120509-01

Ravert, P. (2002). An integrative review of computer-based simulation in the education process. *CIN: Computers, Informatics, Nursing, 20*(5), 203–208. Retrieved from http://search.ebscohost.com/login.aspx?direct=true&db=rzh&AN=2002159431&site=ehost-live

Rodgers, B. L. (2005). *Developing nursing knowledge: Philosophical traditions and influences.* Philadelphia, PA: Lippincott Williams & Wilkins.

Rosen, M. A., Hunt, E. A., Pronovost, P. J., Federowicz, M. A., & Weaver, S. J. (2012). In situ simulation in continuing education for the health care professions: A systematic review. *Journal of Continuing Education in the Health Professions, 32*(4), 243–254. doi:10.1002/chp.21152

Tiffen, J., Corbridge, S., Shen, B. C., & Robinson, P. (2011). Patient simulator for teaching heart and lung assessment skills to advanced practice nursing students. *Clinical Simulation in Nursing, 7*(3), e91–e97.

Weaver, A. (2011). High-fidelity patient simulation in nursing education: An integrative review. *Nursing Education Perspectives, 32*(1), 37–40. doi:10.5480/1536-5026-32.1.37

Weinger, M. (2010). The pharmacology of simulation: A conceptual framework to inform progress in simulation research. *Simulation in Healthcare: The Journal of the Society for Simulation in Healthcare, 5*, 8–15. doi:10.1097/SIH.0b013e3181c91d4a

Wilson, R. D., & Hagler, D. (2012). Through the lens of instructional design: Appraisal of the Jeffries/National League for Nursing Simulation Framework for use in acute care. *Journal of Continuing Education in Nursing, 43*(9), 428–432. doi:10.3928/00220124-20120615-27

Yeung, E., Dubrowski, A., & Carnahan, H. (2013). Simulation-augmented education in the rehabilitation professions: A scoping review. *International Journal of Therapy & Rehabilitation, 20*(5), 228–236. Retrieved from http://search.ebscohost.com/login.aspx?direct=true&db=rzh&AN=2012127287&site=ehost-live

Yuan, H. B., Williams, B. A., & Fang, J. B. (2012). The contribution of high-fidelity simulation to nursing students' confidence and competence: A systematic review. *International Nursing Review, 59*(1), 26–33. doi:10.1111/j.1466-7657.2011.00964.x